S0-AFU-047

A SHEARWATER BOOK

Diagnosis: Mercury

Diagnosis: Mercury

Money, Politics, and Poison

Jane M. Hightower, MD

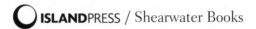
ISLANDPRESS / Shearwater Books

Washington • Covelo • London

A Shearwater Book
Published by Island Press

Copyright © 2009 Jane M. Hightower, MD

All rights reserved under International and Pan-American Copyright
Conventions. No part of this book may be reproduced in any form or by
any means without permission in writing from the publisher: Island
Press, 1718 Connecticut Ave., NW, Suite 300, Washington, DC 20009.

SHEARWATER BOOKS is a trademark of
The Center for Resource Economics.

Library of Congress Cataloging-in-Publication data.

Hightower, Jane M.
Diagnosis mercury : money, politics, and poison /
by Jane M. Hightower.
p.   cm.
Includes bibliographical references and index.
ISBN-13: 978-1-59726-395-5 (cloth : alk. paper)
ISBN-10: 1-59726-395-8 (cloth : alk. paper)
1. Mercury—Toxicology. 2. Mercury wastes—Political aspects 3.
Mercury—Environmental aspects. 4. Mercury—Government policy—
United States. I. Title.
RA1231.M5H54 2009
615.9'25663—dc22   2008022550

British Cataloguing-in-Publication data available.

Printed on recycled, acid-free paper ✪

Manufactured in the United States of America

10   9   8   7   6   5   4   3   2   1

Keywords: mercury, public health, food safety and regulation, fish,
environmental pollution, FDA, EPA, coal-fired power plants,
Iraq seed-grain poisoning, Thimerosal

For my husband Richard,
who knew the dangers of mercury,
and for my boys Luke and Kirk,
for their patient support and wonderful humor.

~ • ~

Contents

Preface

WHEN I FIRST BEGAN TO WRITE a book about mercury and its toxic effects, my goal was to give a broad audience a simple summary of easily understandable information. I hoped to give direction to those with elevated mercury levels and suggest how excess mercury exposure could be avoided while maintaining a healthful diet. I thought I would easily be able to summarize the scientific knowledge acquired from reading the literature. After all, mercury has been known as a poison for centuries, and avoidance of significant exposure seemed so commonsensical. I wondered why we humans had continued to allow ourselves to be exposed to it in significant quantities.

It did not take long to realize that the task of tracking down what lay behind the mercury issue would prove far more challenging than I initially imagined. Wherever I looked—in the scientific literature, in court cases, or in accounts of mercury poisonings in different parts of the world—there were those who thought mercury was toxic at almost any dose and those who thought mercury was not much to worry about except in extreme cases. Those who appeared most certain that mercury typically caused no harm, it seemed, were generally trying to sell a product that contained mercury or had connections to an industry that bellowed it into the air or dumped it into the water.

As a practicing physician of internal medicine, I at first felt obligated to find answers for patients who had elevated blood levels of mercury and appeared to have been adversely affected by considerable consumption of fish. But as I gathered documents, studied the science, and spoke to key individuals, troubling facts began to emerge. I found that the mercury issue reached well beyond my patients into a tangled thicket of corporate interests, government regulation, international politics, and battles over what consumers had the right to know about what they were eating.

This investigation of mercury and our health was made possible with the help of many individuals and with the support of my family, friends, and colleagues. I sincerely thank my patients for allowing us all to learn from them. I changed the names in this text to protect their identity. For all their technical support over the years, I especially would like to thank Kathryn Mahaffey, U.S. Environmental Protection Agency; Dr. Philippe Grandjean, Harvard University; Lynda Knobeloch, Wisconsin Division of Public Health; and Alan Stern, New Jersey Department of Environmental Protection. Many librarians were invaluable in helping to find rare documents, and I am greatly appreciative. I am especially grateful to Kathy Kimber of the California Pacific Medical Center Library for providing me with the many references I consulted for this book and for her enthusiasm. I am also very appreciative of Michael Bender of Mercury Policy Project for organizing and networking the many individuals involved in the mercury issue at large, and for all of his resourcefulness, and for Shelby Gregory for leading me to the treasure divers and their stones. I truly appreciate the added perspective provided by Frank D'Itri and Aileen Smith, as well as their careful documentation of historical events that involved methylmercury in fish in years past. Last, and most important, I thank my editor, Jonathan Cobb, for all of his direction and expertise in making this book exist for the public.

CHAPTER 1

The Discovery

I HAVE A VIVID MEMORY as a young child in the 1970s of my mother asking me to look in the cupboards and pull out all of the canned tuna she had stored there. Together we checked numbers on the cans to see if they were on a recall list. I didn't know at the time why the cans were being recalled, or even why, really, we were removing the cans from our shelves.

I hadn't thought about that event in decades, not until a few years ago when I found myself trying to make sense of the complaints of a series of patients in my San Francisco medical practice. In the early 1970s the U.S. Food and Drug Administration (FDA) had decided that the amount of mercury in some of the fish then being canned posed a health risk to consumers. The concern died down, so somehow, the fisheries industry must have been able to resolve the problem. Or did it?

~•~

One morning in January 2000, a patient I shall call Toshiko came to see me complaining of an array of puzzling symptoms. A soft-spoken but serious businesswoman of Japanese descent in her mid-forties, Toshiko lived some miles away and traveled the world frequently. On her way back from Japan the previous week, she said she had fainted in the restroom on the plane. She had some nausea but no vomiting and still did not feel well.

Over the next hour I asked Toshiko my usual list of questions as an independent practitioner of internal medicine. This was the second time she had fainted recently, it turned out. And she had other symptoms, too: intermittent stomach upset, headache, fatigue, trouble concentrating, and hair loss.

1

I watched the emotions play across her face as I laid out a plan for the various lab tests and consultations with a neurologist and a cardiologist that I felt would be necessary to obtain an accurate diagnosis. I also gave her a prescription for her upset stomach and a list of tasks she could do that might aid our search for the cause of her symptoms. With that she thanked me, and out the door she went. I hoped she would not be so overwhelmed that she would not return.

At that time, my days consisted of medical consultations based on sometimes hours of independent research. I loved my work as a diagnostician. Often patients would bring stacks of medical records to my office for a second opinion on what their regular doctor had suggested. From local referrals to ones from the Mayo Clinic, I saw many medical workups for a wide variety of complaints and conditions. I had reduced the time I spent at the office after giving birth to twin boys two years prior, but balancing work and home remained an evolving test of fortitude. Recently, I had been encountering a surprising number of patients with multiple complaints for which I could not find the cause.

Oftentimes in medicine, a cause cannot be found for a patient's discomfort. As new technologies are discovered that allow for diagnosis, and better dissemination of information is obtained with the Internet, recognition and cures can now be discovered for many conditions that went previously indeterminate.

Many of the patients for whom I could not find a diagnosis, including Toshiko, had entirely normal results on basic laboratory tests designed to identify the sources of many common problems—from thyroid conditions and menopause to anemia and inherited metabolic disorders. The gastroenterologist did say that a mild gastritis showed up on Toshiko's endoscopy, but, as expected, the cardiologist gave her a clean bill of health. The neurologist also found no cause of her fainting and other symptoms.

Looking at the results of tests I had ordered for a patient was like getting to see if I had solved a mystery, and it was something I really enjoyed. One thing that caught my eye in Toshiko's lab report, though, was the inclusion of results for a test I hadn't ordered: a measure of blood mercury level. And it showed an elevated level of mercury in Toshiko's blood.

The colleague who had ordered the test, a dermatologist named Kathy Fields, was no ordinary clinician. She was an avid researcher and had developed an acne treatment called Proactiv, for which she was frequently seen in television infomercials. When I called her, I jokingly asked what type of acne cream she was using to cause the mercury elevation in my patient. She laughed and quickly explained what had led to the test. She had been traveling in Idaho, she said, when a caller to a public radio station there complained of hair loss ostensibly caused by eating fish from a lake polluted with mercury. Curious, Dr. Fields wanted to test someone with abnormal hair loss herself, so when my patient appeared with that symptom and mentioned that she ate fish regularly, Dr. Fields added the test.

Neither Dr. Fields nor I had experience interpreting the result, so we had no idea whether Toshiko's elevated blood mercury level meant anything significant. Dr. Fields even wondered whether she had ordered the correct test.

I read the report that accompanied Toshiko's lab result carefully. Her whole-blood mercury level was 18.5 micrograms per liter (mcg/l), considerably above normal, defined by the lab as "less than 10.0 mcg/l at the end of a workweek." Fish can have mercury in it, I knew, and my patient consumed fish. But how did "end of a work week" enter in? I was not aware of any occupations that required a person to eat fish or mercury. I gave San Francisco Poison Control a call to sort all this out.

Poison Control was quite responsive to my questions at first. An intern referred me to a regular employee, who then consulted with her team. She called back to say that I needed to repeat the blood mercury test and collect a twenty-four-hour urine test concurrently. She wasn't sure why my patient had an elevated mercury level and suggested I ask the patient to allow her home to be evaluated. We discussed potential sources of exposure, which include mercury/silver dental amalgams (an amalgam being a mix of mercury with another metal), vaccines, herbs, homeopathic remedies, herbicides whose residues remained on fruits and vegetables, well water, cosmetics, and fish.

Mercury is a naturally occurring element, and is commonly seen in instruments such as thermometers and barometers. There are different types of mercury compounds, some of inorganic mercury, some organic mercury; unfortunately, Toshiko's blood test alone would not identify what type she was being exposed to. The several forms of mercury are cleared from the body differently and have different ranges of toxicities and symptoms of overexposure. Without the correct test, an accurate diagnosis may not be possible. Organic mercury, which has carbon atoms attached and is seen in food items, predominantly fish, is excreted in hair, feces, sweat, and breast milk but not to an appreciable degree through the kidneys. Nearly all mercury in fish is a form of organic mercury, methylmercury. Therefore, a blood or hair mercury test is more useful diagnostically in exposure from fish consumption than the routine urine heavy-metal screen used to detect the presence of inorganic mercury that most doctors are taught to order first.

Inorganic mercury has noncarbon atoms attached, and its presence in the environment can be increased by coal-fired power plants that emit mercury into the air and by chlor-alkali plants that dump mercury into the water. Mercury from these sources, whether from pollution or naturally occurring, is converted to methylmercury by bacteria in the soils and water. The bacteria are taken up by small organisms, which are themselves consumed by small crustaceans or fish, which are gobbled up by larger fish, and so on. These creatures do not rid themselves of mercury very well, so mercury becomes increasingly concentrated as you go up the food chain, a process known as bioaccumulation. Environmental scientists have been reporting for many years that high methylmercury exposure has an adverse impact on the development and fertility of many fish and other animals. Of the mercury compounds we humans are commonly exposed to, methylmercury is also deemed the most toxic. This is because it is readily absorbed by the body and has been known to enter every one of the body's cells, binding to tissue sulfhydryl molecules and interacting with other elements.

Within only a couple of days of Toshiko's visit, another new patient with puzzling symptoms came to see me. This time it was a woman in her early fifties, educated, responsive, and athletically svelte. As she took a seat in my consultation room, my office assistant happened to place the day's lab results on my in-box. I glanced down and saw Toshiko's retest results. The repeat blood mercury was essentially the same as the first time, while her urine test did not show an appreciable amount of mercury, indicating that she was being exposed to an organic mercury compound. Could it be the fish she ate? She ate at the finest restaurants and shopped at reputable grocery stores, and she said she did not consume any noncommercial fish while in the United States or Japan. Toshiko's was a puzzling case, as medical school training, when mercury was considered, mostly focused on occupational exposures that involved inhaling elemental or inorganic mercury, hence the laboratory report that defined mercury exposure by one's workweek. That was why physicians were often only taught to order a urine metal-screening test, which would be positive in such cases. I wondered if we physicians had been missing something. I put off thinking further about this and looked over to my new patient, eager to get started, and took my seat.

As soon as I greeted Amy, as I will call her, she declared in utter frustration that her house seemed to be making her sick. She went on to tell me of the waxing and waning nature of her symptoms—fatigue, headache, trouble concentrating, stomach upset, and even hair loss. It was like having a hangover, she said, only she did not drink alcohol. Sometimes she could not get out of bed for a couple of days. When she and her husband stayed at their house in France, she would feel better after a couple of months but would feel ill again within days of returning home to the United States.

She had seen numerous allopathic doctors, alternative care doctors, homeopaths, herbalists, and chiropractors. She had spent a small fortune on scans of her head and abdomen and had numerous tests performed on every body fluid imaginable. This certainly sounded like another I-don't-know-what-you-have case. Still thinking of Toshiko's latest lab report, I wondered to myself if Amy ate fish. I took a deep breath and got down to work.

Physicians have a standard protocol for obtaining information from their patients. We try to do our line of questioning the same way each time so as not to forget any question. We start with the chief complaint, or why the patient is there; followed by the history of the present illness; then past medical, surgical, and psychiatric history; allergies to medications; medications taken; family history; social history; and a review of symptoms for every organ in the body. I listened intently as Amy explained her symptoms in the initial history. When she seemed finished, I asked a simple question: "Do you eat fish?"

No one had asked about her diet before—ever—let alone a particular part of her diet. She looked at me strangely and said tentatively, "Yes." "How often?" She replied in a more stern voice, "I am a vegetarian, so I do not eat meat."

If I had learned anything taking care of people in San Francisco and the rest of the Bay Area, it was to tread carefully around a vegetarian's diet. So I dropped the subject until an appropriate time to ask again arose.

My medical school training was at the University of Illinois at Chicago, one of the first medical school programs to require doctors in training to take a nutrition class. Some students thought the class was a joke; food and nutrition had nothing to do with contracting non-infectious disease unless you were malnourished, they felt. In practice, I soon learned that malnourishment was easier accomplished than once thought, as many people even place themselves on "diets" of various colors—"I don't eat anything white" or "I only eat green." Early in my career one young woman came in with a stack of supplements and complained of not feeling well. She was a vegetarian, she said, but didn't eat vegetables—thus the supplements. What did she eat? "Lean Cuisine," she replied. Ever since, I routinely ask my patients about their diets.

I revisited the issue with Amy by asking her to tell me about the role of fish in her diet. She had been consuming fish at least nine times a week—tuna, swordfish, sushi, sea bass, halibut, and, as she put it, "you know, all kinds of fish." Little did she or I know then that her "variety" consisted of fish with the highest mercury content sold in the commercial market. Along with the other labs I ordered, I included a test for blood mercury level. Hers was 26.0 mcg/l, considerably higher than the

18.5 mcg/l found in Toshiko's blood. And the urine test? Mercury was not found.

Once I began to test patients for mercury's presence in instances where it seemed warranted, I soon found I had an increasing number with elevated levels on my hands. They had come to me for a variety of reasons, including nonspecific symptoms of headache, stomach upset, fatigue, insomnia, joint and muscle pain, hair loss, trouble concentrating, and the like. Some just came to establish me as their primary care physician and had no evident symptoms but were avid consumers of fish. The symptoms among individuals who had them could have come from a variety of sources—from viral illnesses to cancers—but I began finding that mercury seemed to be implicated in many instances. In my training, I remembered hearing from my professors that mercury can stay in the body "forever." Well, forever can be a very long time. Surely, my best internal medicine textbook would help me with my many questions. How long does it really stay in the body? Is long-term exposure harmful? And how can its level in the body be significantly reduced?

I began to search for information. My patients were being exposed to mercury through their fish consumption, it seemed. Since fish mercury is in the form of methylmercury, I first looked up methylmercury in the *Cecil Textbook of Medicine*, a standard general text most physicians would have on their shelf. There was only one paragraph devoted to methylmercury. The milder symptoms of methylmercury were said to be the same as for elemental mercury (commonly known as quicksilver, the type of mercury found in a thermometer): insomnia, nervousness, mild tremor, impaired judgment and coordination, decreased mental efficiency, emotional lability, headache, fatigue, loss of sex drive, and depression. There were also more severe symptoms listed: severe paresthesias (a prickling or tingling sensation of the skin), trouble speaking, trouble walking, tunnel vision, hearing loss, blindness, microcephaly (small brain size at birth), spasticity, paralysis, and coma. The "reference range"—what is considered the maximum acceptable to maintain good health—was less than 50 mcg/l for whole blood. No further information as to diagnosis, treatment, prognosis, and so forth was included in the textbook.[1]

Perhaps it was just that my 1992 edition was out of date, so I looked on the Internet and came across a 1998 report to Congress about mercury written by the Environmental Protection Agency (EPA). I combed its volumes of pages extensively, hungry for information for my patients. The report recommended that the mercury level for humans be less than 5 mcg/l in order to avoid adverse health effects, especially with exposure over a lifetime—that was one-tenth what my medical text said was acceptable. Toshiko's level exceeded the EPA recommendation by a factor of more than three, and Amy's level was more than five times what was recommended. For me, a particularly fascinating part of the report was the comment that those who chose large predatory fish to eat could be at risk for significant mercury exposure.[2] The EPA seemed to know that patients like Amy and Toshiko existed, but how could I make sense of the discrepancies between the two sources in order to advise my patients well?

The FDA, whose responsibility was to monitor the mercury levels and other contaminants in fish, had a Web site that contained only a cursory advisory about methylmercury in fish, aimed mainly at pregnant women, which said to limit swordfish. Some of my fish-loving patients ate swordfish, but many did not. Information as to what human blood mercury level was considered safe or harmful was not found on the FDA web site.

From my reading of the medical literature, there was no known use for mercury of any kind in the human body, so shouldn't the normal mercury level for humans be close to zero? I read once that even if you ate common dirt, your mercury level should not be greater than 2 mcg/l unless you were in an unusually contaminated area. Committees of scientists, including those at the FDA, are usually involved with establishing standards for laboratory test reporting. The thought that a bit of mercury in one's blood was okay as long as it was less than 10 mcg/l, as the lab report for Toshiko's blood test indicated, just seemed wrong.

I called Poison Control again and was assigned a toxicology fellow. He sounded quite interested in what I had found among my patients, and I told him that I wanted to conduct a systematic survey on my patient population. Since this was a toxicologist-in-training, I thought he might be interested in helping with such an endeavor and publishing a paper with me. We spoke about the EPA's mercury report and discussed a strategy for setting up a study. At his request, I sent him some papers and abstracts; he said he wanted to meet with me after he looked at them. I also e-mailed him—several times. But I never heard from him again.

I continued with the survey on my own, as I had developed a list of questions I thought relevant and standardized my interview routine. I did not know what I would find or where it would lead. I knew that there could be serious consequences of mercury in large doses, but there was little systematic information on what happened with chronic low-level exposures. And what constituted a "significant" level of exposure, as the EPA used the term in its mercury report? It all seemed so vague.

As for how the environment and its now numerous added chemicals relate to a person's health, I was initially lost in the same abyss as my patients. Although medical school included some subjects in occupational medicine, it did not cover the environmental exposures that the general public would most likely encounter. As physicians we depended on government agencies to tell us if there was a recall for some item or if exposure to a particular source would place our patients at risk for adverse effects and disease. The general attitude among my colleagues was, "If the FDA isn't worried about something, why should we be?"

I called Poison Control a couple more times, as I discovered additional patients with elevated mercury levels; some of their blood levels, I was discovering in the literature, were higher than those of people in other countries already being studied for the effects of mercury exposure. I called patients at home and on their cells, asking them, "What's for dinner?" Poison Control was undoubtedly getting tired of hearing from me. I was the only physician identifying multiple people with elevated mercury levels. I had the horrifying thought that I was walking the top of the fence between the image of a nutter and that of an academically concerned physician.

I would need to become overwhelmingly competent in this subject, I soon realized, if anyone was to take me seriously. Perhaps I was just making too much of this, I'd worry; but then a new patient with an elevated mercury level would come in. No professional I had spoken to could help me sort out what the elevated mercury levels of my patients meant, let alone what to tell them. In the initial discovery, mercury was not on my colleagues' radar screens. When I asked some of them to test some of their own patients, they typically listened calmly to my concerns, then proceeded without further apparent thought on the matter. After all, the literature, FDA, and EPA did not provide a consistent directive for us. Poison Control eventually referred me to the state public health department for advice on how to manage my mercury-exposed patients.

In my search for information, I had already called many people, such as those in public health in surrounding communities, communicable disease specialists, epidemiologists, and other physicians. I even met with our hospital's chief residents to see if they would be interested in writing a paper with me to report the findings of my patient survey. I envisioned that they would share my enthusiasm and idealism, but the meeting proved an exercise in futility.

The Marin County public health representative was quite interested at first, especially since the San Francisco Bay Area has one of the highest breast cancer rates in the nation. I asked if there were any reports of high blood-mercury levels in his jurisdiction. I couldn't be the only physician who was noticing this problem, I thought. He read parts of the *Mercury Study Report to Congress* on my suggestion and seemed genuinely concerned—until he spoke to a California state "seafood specialist," who insisted that my patients got their mercury from perfumes and cosmetics. Of course, my male patients did not accept this explanation and laughed at the specialist's ignorance and insensitive declaration.

Trying to get to anyone in the state government who might know much of anything about mercury was a challenge. I finally made my way up the phone ladder and spoke to a woman who said she was a research scientist at the California Department of Public Health, Alyce Ujihara. She and I discussed the blood levels I was seeing in my patients, and she said she would speak to her director, who, it seemed, was too busy to speak to me.

A few days later, I called again. Ms. Ujihara informed me this time that a blood mercury level of up to 200 mcg/l was okay in adults. I was incredulous. Was she sure of this? She had checked with her director, she said, who stated this as fact. A level of 200 mcg/l was four to ten times higher than what I was seeing in my patients and forty times the ceiling recommended by the EPA's report. "Much of the information we have as to mercury exposures comes from poisonings, such as the Iraq methylmercury seed grain poisoning of 1971," she went on.

It was an offhand remark, and I didn't pursue it then, but it caught my attention. In my training, I had heard of two major mercury poisonings, one that took place in Iraq, the other in Japan. Because the incidents seemed too horrific to ever happen again, little was said in the medical school literature about them.

I asked Ms. Ujihara if she was familiar with the *Mercury Study Report to Congress*. She was, and she recalled its recommendation that blood mercury levels be kept to less than 5 mcg/l to protect infants and children, sensitive people, and people likely to experience repeated exposure over a lifetime. She hesitated, and in spite of her department's discordant advice, admitted that there was no minimal dose known that was safe, nor did anyone know for how long one could be exposed without negative health effects.

That same week, the San Francisco Public Health epidemiologist, Rajiv Bhatia, MD, readily accepted an invitation to come to my office to see what was going on, and to share information he had on the chemicals that lurked in the San Francisco Bay. He was an expert on bay fish and their exposure to extensive amounts of pollutants, mercury included. In our meeting, I explained that none of my patients had consumed fish directly out of the bay, but instead were getting their fish from commercial sources such as the grocery stores and restaurants.

After Dr. Bhatia left, I called the Marin Marine Mammal Center. There had been a beaching of whales in Pacifica the previous week. If my patients were eating commercial fish from the region and getting high doses of mercury, I wondered if the whales could be affected by the same source. I spoke to one of the veterinarians and explained that I was seeing an increase in blood mercury levels in my patients who ate fish. I asked whether the mercury levels of the beached whales were being tested. "The whales that are predatory can have extremely high mercury levels," he said. "They tolerate it very well."

"The whales are on the beach—aren't they supposed to be swimming in the water?" I replied. It didn't look like they were tolerating anything well. He then said they were "doing some tests" but did not tell me what they were testing for.

When I got off the phone, I concluded that it was best for me to stick to humans. I was having enough trouble figuring out how this poison was affecting some of my patients—better not take on the whales' problem, too. In fact, the mercury issue, I was realizing, was a lot bigger than I had thought. It was showing up in many different places. How did so much of it come to be in the ocean in the first place that there were such large concentrations in fish? The mercury was getting there somehow—was it related to mercury from coal-fired power plants that was sometimes in the news? If any significant contribution were from some polluting industry, wouldn't the government be trying to stop it? After all, the protein and nutrients in fish could be important for good health, and fishing was big business.

There is nothing worse, for both patient and doctor, than a medical condition that no one really understands. From recognition to diagnosis to treatment, patients want answers and resolutions to their health issues. It is one thing to diagnose a rare but recognized disease or to identify something new; it is understood in such cases that not much may be known about the condition or how to treat it. But mercury is a very old, known poison. Paradoxically, although it seemed controversial, few in the medical world were apparently concerned. Perhaps it was just too complicated, with not enough consensus on what to do.

But then I would come back to my patients again. People with high mercury levels in their blood really seemed to be affected adversely, and their exposure seemed to involve a common and important food, a food that, if one believed the ads, was "heart healthy," "nutritious," and "essential." I was puzzled, too, that the EPA had a clear recommendation for a safe maximum blood mercury level, but the FDA apparently did not. Perhaps the FDA did not know that people like my patients existed. As a physician, I felt a responsibility to bring to the attention of others an adverse drug or food reaction that wasn't being noticed. I went into internal medicine because I loved the puzzle-solving aspect of doctoring. Intrigued, I just had to know more. At the time, though, I had no inkling of how much I would learn about the politics of mercury, how extensive the problem of mercury was in the world, the extent of corporate interests in the issue, or the kind of attention my patients would get.

CHAPTER 2

Finding My Way

A S MORE MERCURY RESULTS FROM MY PATIENTS CAME IN, and those with relatively high levels described how their symptoms were adversely affecting their everyday lives, I kept reading as much as I could about mercury and health. Resolving the issue of whether my patients' symptoms were caused by mercury in their blood would take a thorough investigation.

I was known by many of my colleagues as a physician who had a penchant for sorting out unusual or difficult cases. My patients, therefore, were typically referrals from other physicians or from my existing patients. I took care of those with evident health problems, as well as those who wanted preventive or "primary" care. I always had a waiting list for new patients, though I was neither a participating provider for any health care plan nor listed in the Yellow Pages. Most of my patients were upper middle class and higher in economic status, college educated, and health conscious. The majority were white, and the rest were Hispanic, Asian, black, and of mixed race or ethnicity. A natural question was why I had so many patients with a mercury problem. At first, I wasn't sure myself. Fish consumption, as well as elevated mercury levels, was certainly a common denominator. Perhaps it was something else in the fish that caused the symptoms I was finding? In any case, mercury was associated with fish consumption and was easy to follow in the blood, and those associations were promising paths to pursue.

Four months after my first mercury patient was discovered, I spoke to my friend Kathy Fields again. I told her of the vast array of symptoms patients with high levels of mercury in their blood had complained of and that after a few months off fish, they typically said they felt noticeably better. Some of these patients had had their symptoms for more than a year, some for more than three years. Nearly all of their complaints, it turned out, came after they had increased their consumption of large, predatory fish—tuna, swordfish, sea bass, and the like. Often, their dietary change came about after some life-changing event—such as a new job, a move to the area, or a marriage—had brought a higher income or more accessibility to those fish.

Since Kathy had close ties to the press, she thought I should go to her contacts with what I was already finding among my patients—given the seriousness of the problem and its general lack of recognition. Medical and scientific journal editors explicitly ask authors not to release data to the press before scientific publication. But when public health was at risk, the doctor or scientist had an obligation to notify the public of a potential hazard. So I decided to make public the mercury levels I was finding in a set of patients and the similarity of their complaints, and then to report that information to the FDA. I knew about the patients I saw as one physician, but I could not predict how prevalent this mercury problem was in our community or throughout the country and abroad.

A freelance writer and former prosecuting attorney, Patricia Steele, also phoned me after hearing of my patients' mercury levels from Dr. Fields. Steele had been working with San Francisco's Channel 4 (KRON) news as a journalist and producer. I explained the levels of mercury I had recently discovered in about fifteen of my patients and the array of their symptoms that appeared to be related to the elevated mercury levels in their blood and hair. We realized that in the Bay Area a significant number of people consumed large predatory fish regularly. Those fish not only contained more mercury, but they were also more expensive to harvest and to buy. At first we thought about the more affluent people in the Bay Area, who dined at fine restaurants and bought fish in the finest fish markets, though that did not stop them from indulging in canned tuna, sometimes frequently. They tended not to like bones in their fish or a fishy flavor, and they were not deterred by price. The seafood combo they ordered at the restaurant was not the fried cod, shrimp, and clam chowder more common to people in other parts of the country, but was instead swordfish, ahi, and sea bass.

Whatever tuna sushi or albacore tuna they consumed at lunch or dinner also contributed to their mercury dose. It was not until later that I learned we had plenty of company across the nation and around the world.

I was already concerned about the discrepancy I had discovered between the standards of the FDA and the EPA on just how much mercury was safe to consume, and what a safe level was in one's blood. There was a standard for maximum safe blood mercury levels that lurked in the shadows of FDA advisories that was mentioned to me by various experts, but not easily confirmed through literature and Internet searches. This level for adults was 200 mcg/l. But to add to the confusion, the FDA was in charge of overseeing commercial fish, while the EPA was in charge of noncommercial, or sport, fish. I was especially confused and a bit amused to learn that in some cases the consumption advisories of the two agencies actually differed for the same species of fish.

The agencies' advice on what was an acceptable mercury level in a liter of a person's blood differed by about 195 micrograms (mcg). That may not sound like a lot, but it was huge in its implications for consumption. It was the difference between consuming two-thirds of a single 6-ounce can (4 ounces of albacore) per week versus about twenty-eight cans (168 ounces) for a 132-pound person. The discrepancy posed a particular problem when I needed to speak to individual patients about what was safe for them to consume. And then there was yet a third standard, the guidance proffered by the *Cecil Textbook of Medicine*, which declared a blood mercury level of less than 50 mcg/l as the threshold dosage; for the 132-pound individual, that would yield an allowance of seven cans, or 42 ounces, of albacore per week.

By the time Patricia Steele called back, she had researched the mercury issue for her television station by seeking out previous court cases and government documents that involved the regulation of mercury in fish. In the 1970s, she discovered, in order to limit the amount of mercury getting into the people, the FDA had to decide how much mercury would be allowed in the fish sold commercially. The amount of mercury in fish tissue is measured in mcg/g or parts per million (ppm). At that time, the FDA had raised the allowable mercury concentration in fish from 0.5 mcg/g to 1 mcg/g, double the EPA's allowance. She also had spoken to Michael Bender, who had cofounded an organization called the Mercury Policy Project. He had attended many meetings with government and nongovernment agencies and was following the mercury issue closely. According to him, swordfish, ahi, and shark were no longer being monitored for mercury content by the FDA or EPA, even though 36 percent of swordfish, 33 percent of shark, and 4 percent of ahi had mercury concentrations over 1 mcg/g, the FDA "action level" above which those fish should not be offered for sale. This "action level," I learned, was not really enforceable, as there was wide variability among individual fish, even within a species, and the FDA did not have the time or the resources to test every fish that would be going to the market. Therefore, certain species of large predators were sold with mercury levels higher than 1 mcg/g without any warning to the consumer.

Patricia wanted to test the mercury levels in a sample of fish from local grocery stores and asked me how much the test would cost. Although I didn't know how much a fish tissue test cost, my patients had been getting their blood mercury tests done for $5.46. I had been curious about this, as it seemed an error in billing. I was entertained when patients reported that they had been told in the lab that the test was unusual and might not be covered by their insurance. This was probably the cheapest test I had ever ordered and it is run on the same machine a blood lead level is run on. By contrast, the charge for a thyroid function test was more than $100. Maybe the insurance companies needed to get into the fish debate. A simple, cheap test for mercury, done at the beginning of the workup for those at risk, and simple dietary advice could have saved the companies thousands of dollars with the first fifteen of my mercury patients alone.

Patricia and her team's ability to put a story together on short notice was impressive, and her story aired June 29, 2000, on our local KRON 4 news. My husband's parents came for dinner that night, and we all watched together. My two boys, who were two years old, wanted to know how I got into the TV.

Within twenty-four hours, I began getting telephone calls from people wanting to come in for evaluation of their mercury levels and fish consumption. It was not the flood that one might have expected but a steady stream that seemed to get more intense every day.

Through Patricia Steele, I met the lead author of the 1998 *Mercury Study Report to Congress*, Kathryn Mahaffey, one of the world's most knowledgeable people on the toxicity of mercury and the assessment of risk to the public. She was director of the Health Hazards Assessment Division of the EPA in Washington, DC. Surprising to me, Katy, as I came to know her, answered her own phone when I called. I was therefore able to tell her directly about the survey of my patients' diets, health histories, and subsequent mercury levels. She was quite interested and said that the EPA knew that such a subpopulation existed but did not know how prevalent it was.

I asked her why there was such a discrepancy between EPA and FDA standards on how much mercury one could consume safely. She sidestepped the question but suggested I read two reports that would soon be released. She could not discuss them in detail as they were "embargoed" until their official publication dates, but she said that the first report, from the National Academy of Sciences, would be out the following month and included discussion of the EPA's reference dose. The second, from the Centers for Disease Control, and scheduled to be released in the next four months, would be on mercury levels reported in the National Health and Nutrition Examination Survey (NHANES), a nutrition survey that was supposed to be representative of the U.S. population as a whole.

The EPA's mercury reference dose of 0.1 mcg per kg of body weight per day is the threshold dose of mercury that can be consumed without doing harm, in the agency's view. An uncertainty factor of ten was included in the equation in figuring out this dose, to account for sensitivity among individuals, fish mercury levels, and unforeseen factors.

My depth of knowledge on this subject was embarrassingly shallow, to the point that I did not even know what to ask Katy when I spoke with her. She was certainly concerned about the issue, though, and encouraged me to document what I was seeing in my practice. She also referred me to ABC's *20/20* program. The program's producers wanted to cover the mercury-in-fish issue, she said, and she knew they were looking for doctors with patients who might have been adversely affected by mercury.

In the end, Katy reassured me that my population and survey were important and encouraged me to make them my charge. After I hung up, I just sat for a moment, took a deep breath, and thought about my "charge." Although I was learning fast, I knew I had a long way to go before I really understood enough to guide my patients through the maze of contradictory reports on mercury effects and advise them on finding appropriate consultants that could help sort out their symptoms and other health complaints.

I was frustrated by how little I had been able to find out so far about the levels of methylmercury that affected a population. It was only when my brother, a longtime hunter and fisherman, showed me his California Department of Fish and Game brochure that I discovered that advisories were listed for noncommercial fish. That was interesting, as some fish in the grocery stores and restaurants had higher mercury levels than what was listed as safe for fishermen. Where was the FDA booklet? Come to find out, there was none.

I hadn't been able to get advice from Katy on how to address my patient's mercury levels. But then, the EPA was in the public health sector, where risk assessments are made for populations, not for specific individuals. I was looking for answers to relay to my patients. Do you just stop mercury ingestion and then recover automatically, or do you need a medication or other form of treatment to remove the mercury from the body?

My alternative care colleagues were known to give their patients a substance called a chelator, which would ostensibly remove "toxins"— including mercury—from the body. When I inquired about this treatment among the clinicians who prescribed it, however, I discovered that they had not conducted any scientific study that would justify their approach. Therefore, whether chelation for this level of mercury exposure was necessary or whether it in itself caused harm, was unknown.

If my patients' nonspecific symptoms arose from methylmercury exposure, surely similar cases had to have been reported before, and I thought I might be able to learn something from them. On the Internet I did find a recent paper from the Wisconsin Bureau of Public Health about a family exposed to methylmercury through the consumption of sea bass.[1] In that paper, one of the adults complained of sleep disturbances and concentration difficulties. This was my only clue that I was on the right track.

By June I was following about thirty people with elevated mercury levels. I also began to reconsider the ailments of one of my earlier patients—I'll call her Sally—a lovely woman and quite health conscious. Her previous consultants had given her the diagnosis of chronic fatigue, but it hadn't seemed quite right. Now I recalled that in 1995 her previous doctor, an alternative care physician, had measured her hair mercury level. At that time, I didn't know how to evaluate her level of 5.08 mcg/g. I ordered a twenty-four-hour urine collection for mercury, not aware that the test would indicate exposure only to inorganic mercury, not methylmercury. When it came back "normal," we simply did not proceed further. Now it was the year 2000, and Sally was still symptomatic. I called her to reinvestigate her mercury level, inquire about her diet, and conduct my survey of her diet and symptoms. I faxed her a lab slip to have her blood mercury tested, and we set up a follow-up appointment. She came in the day the results of her blood test arrived.

Our conversation encompassed what I had learned about the mercury in her blood, and I explained that from her report, I noticed that she had been consuming a lot of fish that were high in mercury such as swordfish, sea bass, and ahi and also medium- and low-mercury fish in large quantities. "Oh, yes, I love fish," she said. "It's so good for you. I also have a high metabolism and eat large portions for my small body. I've never had a weight problem." When I asked again about her symptoms, she responded, "I get fatigue that seems to come in waves. I get an upset stomach sometimes, but I have not been able to attribute it to anything. My body aches all over, and I feel that I am losing my memory and my hair." Had she ever had trouble with concentration or thinking? "I feel like I am in a fog sometimes," she responded. "I feel like I am thinking through a box of Kleenex." Foggy thinking was such a common description of my mercury-affected patients that I later began calling the syndrome "fish fog."

The mercury concentration in her blood was 76 mcg/l, I told her, which was very high by the EPA's standard, somewhat elevated by the measures of Cecil's textbook, and not a problem according to the state public health department. I now knew enough to be able to explain in lay terms what her hair mercury level of 5.08 mcg/g, obtained in 1995, meant by comparison. By multiplying her hair level (in mcg/g) by four, one could estimate her blood level in 1995 to be about 20.32 mcg/l if her diet was consistent. Now in 2000, she had a mercury blood concentration more than three times higher. Mercury has a relatively long half-life in the body—about two months on average, which meant that if she stopped consuming methylmercury immediately, her blood level might be 38 mcg/l in two months, though in some individuals, this half-life was much longer, and in some, shorter.

To see if the mercury level in the blood of my ever-growing number of patients fell when fish consumption ended, I asked them all to stop eating fish for at least six months. Sixty-seven of the patients in the year-long survey I conducted agreed to have periodic mercury tests over those six months, and all but two reduced their mercury levels to less than 5.0 mcg/l. Of those two, one reduced to less than 5.0 after the study was over, when he finally stopped consumption, and the other was lost to follow-up. Nearly all of the patients' symptoms resolved after their levels were reduced to less than 5.0 mcg/l. It was unclear from this small study at what level and how long an exposure it might take for a patient to have permanent damage or symptoms from mercury, but some of the patients with particularly high levels and longer exposure times claimed their memory and mental functioning was never back to their baseline. The gastrointestinal effects also appeared to take longer than some of the other symptoms to recover—anywhere from two months to more than a year.

I felt that the improvement in my patients' symptoms with the reduction in their blood mercury levels was strong evidence that they had been having an adverse mercury reaction and that that should be reported to the FDA. Some patients resumed their previous consumption pattern of large fish after the six-month abstinence period only to have their symptoms resume. I have since had no trouble convincing those patients to keep the mercury levels in their blood less than 5.0 mcg/l by having them stick to fish with the lowest mercury concentration.

Whether the elevated mercury levels were caused by fish consumption was easy to sort out by having the patients serve as their own control group. In other words, I simply had the mercury level of each patient measured over time before and after an intervention. In this case, the intervention was simply to stop the exposure through fish.

By the time the *20/20* people called in July 2000 about my mercury patients, I felt I had some information to share that would be helpful for people to know. I told the producers that I would actively participate in the story if they involved Patricia Steele. After a few days of haggling over Patricia's compensation, they agreed to let her be one of the field producers. To me that was important, as I wanted a local media person I trusted to help me in handling the network press. I did not want the camera looking up the noses of my patients in search of tremors, I told the producers. They assured me they would be sensitive to the patients' needs.

Patricia called the same day the *20/20* producer phoned. Her news anchor from KRON, Pam Moore, had called the FDA personally to ask questions but was unable to get anyone to talk to her about mercury in fish even when she complained that "you are the agency that is supposed to protect the people from bad food." Patricia was working on another story, in which her station had tested fish in the local grocery stores and found some to exceed the FDA's action limit of 1.0 mcg/g.

The FDA was still supporting the notion that the presence of up to 200 mcg/l in the blood was without adverse effects. On its Web site the agency had a cursory advisory on only the largest of the predators—that information was not available at the supermarket or fish counter. The FDA seemed to assume that no one in the United States consumed enough fish for mercury to be of concern.

The EPA, by contrast, though restricted to advice for noncommercial fish, had considerably more stringent guidelines in 2000. In addition to having safe limits for mercury in the blood, it is also useful to have guidelines both for how much mercury a person can safely ingest in a day on average, to keep within those blood guidelines, and on the mercury content of various species of fish, as a guide for how much one can safely eat. The EPA's advisory set a limit on a human's mercury consumption at 0.1 mcg per kilogram of body weight a day without adverse effects. This was to keep consumers from raising their blood mercury chronically over 5 mcg/l. The EPA also established a 1 mcg/g action limit on noncommercial fish and publicized it through U.S. Department of Fish and Game and EPA booklets and Web sites. The agency advised fishermen not to consume fish known to be above 1 mcg/g in certain lakes and streams and even gave an advisory for fish over 0.5 mcg/g.[2]

Early on, when I was new at this issue, it seemed as though every time I mentioned the word "mercury" people began to look for the exits. I wasn't sure why, as it seemed pretty simple to me. If you ate mercury, its level in your body went up. If you stopped, it went down. This was not rocket science. It was not until Dr. James Adams of Los Gatos, California, called after seeing Patricia Steele's 2000 story in the local news about mercury in fish that I realized the road ahead was going to be long. Dr. Adams told me that he had been practicing "mercury-free" dentistry for over a decade. He said that the use of mercury/silver tooth amalgams had divided the dental community and suggested that I and others in the medical profession needed to take into consideration that some patients have that type of mercury exposure as well. I admitted to him that, although I had been gaining some momentum in my efforts to obtain mercury information and educate my patients and colleagues, it had been frustrating. His response was, "Just be aware that if you continue with this issue, you will soon have no friends." I took his warning to heart and began to proceed more cautiously when speaking to my patients and my colleagues.

It had been about nine months since my first mercury patient, Toshiko, had been identified. Colleagues had begun coming forward with news of mercury levels among their patients or their own mercury levels, asking me to make sense of what they were finding. Many liked the fact that I was able to estimate the amount of mercury they were consuming through their reported fish consumption and body weight and thereby predict their blood mercury level. Making calculations on mercury and dosing therefore became an every-day experience.

For better or ill, I began to be known for this work around the hospital. Some physicians seemed to avoid me as a result; others engaged me in conversation. I could be anywhere—the hall, the intensive care unit, the lunch table—and be asked to field a mercury question or need to get out my prescription pad and calculator to estimate someone's blood mercury level. By this time, I had memorized all the average mercury levels of fish species on the FDA and EPA tables. One time in a media interview, I got my calculator out and put it on the table. The technician who was placing the microphone asked what it was for. I told her that I wanted to be prepared in case I got nervous when asked to calculate something and could not do it in my head. She gave me a frightened look and exclaimed, "If I had to use a calculator on national television, I would freak!"

Some colleagues didn't hesitate to rib me for my newfound interest, and I usually enjoyed their colorful comments. One of our doctors, Dr. Lory Wiviott, known for his sarcasm and quick wit, asked if it was okay to drive a Mercury. Referring to electronic switches that contained mercury, I told him, "Yeah, as long as you don't eat the switches in the dash."

Patricia eventually got an FDA official in Washington, DC, to speak to her. She explained that people in our area were experiencing high mercury levels from eating fish obtained from restaurants and grocery stores, and that her TV station had found some tuna and swordfish to be over the FDA safe level. The official's response: "Not too many people eat this fish, must be a local problem. It is going extinct anyway."

Clearly, the FDA was not notifying consumers about the mercury content of popular fish such as swordfish, ahi, albacore, and sea bass. When Patricia asked why the agency had discontinued efforts to regulate the amount of mercury in fish sold in grocery stores and restaurants, the FDA spokesperson told her that they stick by their science and that there will be no changes to their reports.

I was not sure which reports they were referring to. The FDA Web site, circa 1995, had not been changed since, and was not extensive when it came to mercury.[3] Perhaps the agency was in the process of issuing another report? In any case, we could not get any opinion from the FDA about how to address the health concerns of patients with elevated mercury levels. That only stirred my curiosity further, as I wondered why there was such an adversarial attitude. I had expected a more collegial atmosphere. Who was making decisions on how much mercury was allowed in commercial fish and how much one could consume, anyway? The FDA Web page did advise consumers to limit the amount of swordfish they ate, but who looked on the Internet every time fish was served just to see if it was safe? What other food items did we need to look up on the Internet to determine their safety? The FDA was supposed to be looking out for the public's safety, but was it? I wasn't sure.

CHAPTER 3

The Media Meets the Victims

B Y AUGUST OF 2000, the *20/20* producers Joan Martelli and Caroline Noel began their descent on my fish-loving patients and me. The producers spoke of filming a whole room full of people suffering from mercury exposure. I cautioned that among my patients were professionals, CEOs, and business owners, and that they might not be eager to go on national TV to tell everyone they were having trouble thinking or remembering. How would the producers feel if they heard their own physician or investment banker saying such things? Aside from one of our local stories going national, the *20/20* production would be the first time the issue would hit a prime-time, nationally syndicated program. The producers began rethinking what they could expect from us.

When I sent letters to my patients offering them a chance to give their opinion about the mercury issue on national television, the idea got mixed reviews. Many just did not want to do it. Many were worried that they would be criticized for consuming too much fish or doing something else wrong, or that they would be ridiculed in the public eye. I told them that I felt they had valid concerns, that I might not want to do it either in their position. I had my own reservations—being the physician to bring this problem to national attention was a responsibility I did not take lightly.

Several weeks went by as the *20/20* people researched their story. Shortly before it was time for them to fly to California, Caroline Noel called. Were any other doctors testing their patients for mercury? She was concerned that I seemed to be the only one. "There must be other doctors who know this," she speculated. "You must be a magnet for these people."

My gut churned as I realized I might be standing on my own on this one. After thinking for a moment, I just stated again the facts of the mercury findings among my patients. "I thought the whole idea of doing the show was to bring to public attention a problem that few seemed to know about," I said. The producers now gave me the impression that because they could not find any other doctor who had been testing for mercury, or knew anything about it, either I was a very odd doc or I had very odd patients. Perhaps both.

I began to ask other physicians if they would test more of their patients who fit the criteria of symptoms like those I had identified or whose blood mercury levels were likely to be over the EPA guideline because of the amount and type of fish they ate. I tried to teach them how to estimate a person's mercury level based on diet, so they could have a rule of thumb for whom to test. Although my colleagues have all been trained in calculating doses of medications based on the size of an individual, mercury math seemed to be cumbersome to many of them. In reply, the obstetricians typically said things like "You can't do anything about it anyway." Or "I do not want to deal with patient anxiety about this." I felt so strongly about the effects of mercury I was seeing as a clinician in a number of my patients that I knew there had to be many others out there with this problem. I would endure what it took to bring this issue into mainstream medicine, I vowed to myself. I asked my patients every question I could think of, from past to present medical, surgical, and psychiatric histories. They also brought with them all records from their prior consultants and past workups.

The news spread at the hospital that *20/20* was preparing to do a story on mercury and would be interviewing my patients and me. My colleagues began to realize my predicament, and many began reading some of the literature themselves. At lunch in the dining room one surgeon spoke about a small tremor he had that was fleeting and said that he had not been feeling well. He estimated that he ingested at least ten times more mercury a month than he should. I and the four other doctors at my table then looked over at Dr. Wiviott, known for eating a pile of albacore tuna on his salad every day and asked how he was feeling. He laughed and responded, "We can thank the hospital chief of staff for the daily tuna. The budget is tight."

More and more physicians began calling me about their own mercury levels as well as their patients'. Some were seeing the same assortment of symptoms as I was. I tried to recruit them to interview with the media, but they felt they did not know enough about the subject to take on questions of the media, the government, and the fishing industry. They responded typically with "I will leave that part to you, Jane!"

Pam Moore and Patricia Steele came to my office again in August to do a follow-up story. This time the interview was more pointed and lasted for an hour. Pam began with "Don't you think you are off on a crusade?" I was only confirming what had been known for some time, that there was mercury in fish and some people could not tolerate it, I explained.

Pam likened the situation to that around the discovery of AIDS. She asked if I were angry with the government because its standards for mercury toxicity seemed to be inadequate. "I would be angry if I were pregnant and eating fish with high mercury," I replied. "As a doctor, though, I have to think scientifically and keep my cool, carefully documenting and watching closely. The EPA was doing its job when it came to noncommercial fish, but the FDA was in charge of standards for commercial fish. I am not on a crusade, just trying to make people better, and if people who have been sick for a long time, some greater than eight years, who have tried many treatments and gone to numerous doctors, get better by decreasing a poison in their body, then perhaps this means something. Only time will tell."[1]

Patricia and her crew attended a press conference that same week where FDA commissioner Jane Henney, MD, spoke. Patricia asked Dr. Henney why the FDA had not publicized or warned pregnant women about mercury levels in fish. Dr. Henney countered that the agency had widely publicized its advice that expectant mothers should not eat swordfish and ahi steaks more than once a month.

This surprised Patricia, and others in the audience, as well; she had not encountered anyone who knew of such warnings or felt that a mention buried on an FDA Web site constituted wide publicity. When

Patricia tried to follow up with further questions, she told me, Dr. Henney made a quick and awkward exit.

Other local media were also weighing in on the mercury debate that August. A patient reported that she had called Dr. Dean Edell, a local TV doctor, on air to ask what a friend who had a very high mercury level should do. Dr. Edell apparently responded that you could eat all the fish you wanted; mercury was not of concern. The person in question was reported to have a blood mercury level of 89 mcg/l—considerably above even the reference range given in Cecil's textbook. Dr. Edell's response did not go over well with Pam Moore and her staff. Pam and Patricia felt that Edell had challenged their reputations and, furthermore, was giving uninformed medical advice. Also, Patricia told me, the EPA press office seemed to be forbidding Dr. Mahaffey to speak in an interview.[2]

So the FDA was running and the EPA was apparently closemouthed, leaving the media to battle out the issue over the airwaves. In the meantime, those who were being adversely affected by mercury were discovering the cause of their symptoms and becoming increasingly frustrated by the government's silence and inaction. I wondered where the scientists were in this debate.

I called the University of California at San Francisco's (UCSF's) Occupational and Environmental Health clinic to ask if they had had any mercury patients. If they did, they might have toxicologists experienced with this issue and could assist me in how to advise my patients. I introduced myself and was kindly transferred to the head nurse for the clinic. I explained that I was conducting a survey of patients' fish intake and mercury levels, and she responded tersely that they had received numerous calls from patients reporting blood mercury levels of only 5.0 to 5.5 mcg/l and wanting advice. She went on to complain, "News magazine people and media sensationalize everything."

I told her that I was not aware of any sensational mercury stories lately; our local channel 4 was trying to be informative. When she came back with "There will be people who panic about this. We need to educate the public and our peers," I tried to allay her fears and told her that at least we agreed that education was in order.

I appreciated her honesty, and since she ran the clinic at that facility, it gave me insight as to how some others in the field might have been thinking. As a physician, I have to tell people news they do not want to hear every day. Just because people are unhappy with what they hear does not mean you don't tell them; especially in California, where the right to know is demanded and is the law of the land.

I then called the Stanford University doctor and professor of medicine who had performed a mercury test on one of the patients I had consulted on. The patient's mercury level had gone from 38 mcg/l to 89 mcg/l some months later. This was the patient on whose behalf a friend had called Dr. Edell. The Stanford doctor exclaimed, "The 89 was probably not accurate, so I discounted it; the 38 was not very high."

According to the charts of mercury content in fish, a reading of 89 would be consistent with the patient's diet of large fish, predominantly swordfish steaks, I replied. Why did he think her level was not accurate? I had called the lab where the test had been done and discussed their controls and methods, I said. The lab had repeated the test and confirmed the 89 mcg/l. The professor did not respond to my comment about the lab but instead informed me that mercury was in his area of expertise and that he gave lectures on it. He then said in an incensed way, "I do not have any of my papers with me. I am away from the office. Why are you calling, anyway?" If this was the kind of attitude my mercury patients were running into, I could see why they had been so frustrated. In any case, it was clear I was not gaining any friendships in making such calls.

The 20/20 people, led by Arnold Diaz, a consumer investigative reporter, arrived on August 30 for filming. The producers had rented a room for the interview. When I walked in, I was happy to see Patricia already there. She had met with the fifteen patients who had agreed to participate and introduced them to each other. One patient in particular, herself a doctor, was very apprehensive.

Arnold Diaz walked into the room carrying a black bag, and we were introduced. We shook hands, but he never really made eye contact. He instead looked over my head and announced, "We need a naysayer in all this to stir things up." I told him that I was sure I could find him a few.

He did not seem to hear me and continued to scan the room, seemingly studying his subjects, who were seated in a bandstand type of arrangement, waiting for the interview to begin. Arnold never talked to my patients or acknowledged them. He just stood there, occasionally checking to make sure his face was right. Funny thing, we were all making sure our faces were in order. Everyone was uneasy and concerned whether they would be respected. The patients were professionals, retired people, and business executives. Three were physicians. They came well dressed and ready to tell their side of the story. They came as individuals and did not know what problems had brought the others there. Only I knew. They were sizing Arnold up, as well.

Arnold began with some general questions, such as, "Who among you eats fish? Who among you had a mercury level over the EPA's limit of 5 mcg/l?" All the people raised their hands with both of these questions. He then asked questions such as, "Who knew there was an FDA advisory on mercury and fish? Who had ever been told that there was mercury in fish when it was purchased?" Of course, none of them raised a hand. He then asked each patient about some of the symptoms they had and their feelings about the situation. They were very impressive, as many had thought about what they would say and knew to keep their answers short. One of the patients produced documentaries for a living and was clear that she wanted to have the public educated about this issue. "We were told fish was good for you," she said. "Had I known that there was so much mercury in the fish I was choosing, and that it was affecting my health, I could have made an educated decision and chosen a different variety."

During the break, one of my colleague-patients said she did not think she should be on the show. She felt uncomfortable being placed with a group of patients. Patricia and Caroline reminded her that, unfortunately, she was a patient. They tried to reassure her, mentioned the importance of her presence, and reminded her that there were two other physicians in the group.

The producers finally talked her into continuing with the interview. I understood what she was feeling. Physicians have often been chastised for speaking up, especially when what they say goes against the powers that be. Those who think outside the box or make new discoveries have often been undermined and labeled charlatans, nutters, or activists by those who could be adversely affected economically. Only time would tell how they would be remembered in health history.

After the patients were interviewed, it was my turn. Two chairs were set up face to face. Arnold gave me no way to read what he could be thinking. I got the impression that he did not know the material well and was struggling with my answers. People in the media knew that if they themselves did not understand the subject matter, the public wouldn't, either. They gear the understanding of the program to the level of a twelve-year-old so that the general public would want to watch. I gave him clear and concise but scientific answers, and he kept asking questions like "Aren't you angry that there are no warnings on mercury in fish?" And "How much mercury is there in canned tuna, anyway, and how much can you eat of it?" When I continued to give numerical values in my answers, he stopped the interview and said, "I don't think they can use any of this—too technical and too many numbers. I guess they may have enough of you for something."

After the interview was over, I felt drained. I wasn't sure I had been able to get my points across in a manner that could be deciphered by the public. But more than that, so much talk about how healthy fish was made me think. A number of other foods could have something in them that could be bad for you, I realized. At the personal level, when it came to food in general, my motto became "Just eat everything and not a whole lot of anything."

We could not assume that the government was monitoring everything, nor could we trust that the food industry would disclose potential harm—that was clear. As consumers, we needed to remain alert and careful in our choices. Industry was playing a balancing game with regulatory agencies and the public health for the health of its own economy. This balancing game was also being played out in the press. If health professionals and government agencies could not adequately and succinctly address the issue, then how could the press handle it? How can you have fair news presentations when critical information is lacking? The industry had the upper hand, as it could always come back with "prove it" when it came to health effects, given our society's tendency to put the burden of proof on the consumer.

I also realized from watching the development of various health-related issues that there are gifted scientists under contract with industry who are too often controlled as to what reports they can reveal to the public, or what they are allowed to research in the first place. Well-intentioned industry scientists can lose their jobs if they report something about a product that is not favorable to the company. Grants to universities from industry can also influence what is studied and how, as well as what is included or not included in final reports. For the consumer, perhaps the anecdotal approach of telling a friend or a sympathetic advocacy or educational group about an emerging problem is ultimately the most powerful approach for overcoming the resistance of naysayers and industry scientists who are paid to look only at certain things, and government officials who do not have the power or will to protect the people.

CHAPTER 4

Spreading the News

WHEN I FIRST BEGAN MY STUDY, I thought I would be providing a service to my patients and hopefully provide others with useful information by publishing my survey results. Fish, methylmercury, and patient health were my focal points. How my patients would fit into the larger issues of mercury in the environment and pollution regulation was not on my radar. I wanted to conduct the survey without influence by outside interest groups or any primary or secondary industries that might be affected by my findings, so I tried to keep a relatively low profile beyond my hospital. Except for being taped for a later showing of *20/20*, which was certainly not the stealthy thing to do, I had interviewed only with the local news and given small lectures to our hospital staff at the California Pacific Medical Center in San Francisco, so only a few people knew much about my study. I was a virtual unknown when it came to prominent players in the controversies over mercury and human health.

My survey was an effort to discover what was raising my patient's mercury levels. It was not about saving the ocean, the turtles, or Charlie the Tuna. I just wanted to do my best. I knew that a lot was at stake, but it would not be until the survey was over and published that I understood its impact, since so little attention had been given to anything but extreme effects of mercury toxicity, at doses that were far beyond my patients' levels of exposure.

In mid-August, I had written letters to my congressional representatives, the FDA, and the EPA expressing my concerns about finding elevated blood mercury levels in patients consuming fish. I believed it was important for physicians to report adverse food and drug reactions to the regulating authorities, and our congressional representatives liked to know what was going on in their jurisdiction. I addressed my first letter to U.S. senator Dianne Feinstein, with copies to California's senators and the representatives of my district.[1] When Senator Feinstein wrote back to say she would ask the FDA to comment on my concerns, it gave me hope that a tradition in which doctors reported their concerns still had some recognition. Senator Feinstein wrote to the FDA soon thereafter.[2] The FDA responded to her on December 21, 2000, but, unfortunately, I did not see a copy of the letter for almost two years, until October 2002, when I came across it on the Internet.

In any case, the reply to Feinstein claimed that "the commercial species that contained the highest average amounts of methylmercury —shark and swordfish—were expensive and were consumed relatively infrequently even by people who may be regarded as consumers of those species. For example, the known average consumption for swordfish among consumers of swordfish was once every several months." The letter went on to say that my patients not only must be consuming amounts that considerably exceeded the national averages, they must be doing so on a very steady basis. It continued, "The FDA's existing consumption advisory was developed to help people avoid that kind of consumption," though "we agree with Dr. Hightower that FDA's consumption advisory has not become widely known." The letter closed by saying, "If Dr. Hightower has specific information (e.g., hair or blood methylmercury levels, adverse symptoms) on individuals who have consumed fish, FDA would be very interested in having an opportunity to review this information."[3] Perhaps when dealing with the FDA, one has to refer to the Internet to get one's mail as well as check for mercury advisories.

Perhaps the FDA did not use the telephone, either. Of course, I would have liked to know at the time that the FDA was interested. Perhaps it was a blessing in disguise, though, as it allowed me to continue with my survey, not only without input from industry and nongovernment agencies, but also without input from the FDA. I had never asked for or received a grant, nor was I part of any remotely interested organization other than the medical societies. This was a grassroots effort, for sure.

Among the first groups of colleagues at my hospital to invite me to speak about mercury to their departments were the nutritionists, neurologists, and obstetricians. Many physicians in our community are health conscious and keen on saving the environment and were interested in environmental toxicants in relation to human health, but only if they saw overwhelming evidence in their most respected medical journals. The trouble was, not enough information was making its way into our medical journals.

The obstetricians were more interested than most in the mercury issue, as it was believed, based on reports in the scientific literature, that the fetal brain was vulnerable to methylmercury. Furthermore, the FDA guidelines for toxicity and the fetal scientific literature seemed contradictory on what likely was to be safe. This left the obstetricians in a quandary when addressing the issue with their patients. Their advice could allow a woman to accept dangerously high levels of mercury in her blood during pregnancy, resulting in damage to her fetus, on the one hand, or perhaps lead her to abort a pregnancy out of the possibly unfounded fear of such damage, on the other. The large differences between the mercury advisories of the FDA, with its acceptable blood mercury pegged at 200 mcg/l, and the EPA, with its acceptable level pegged at 5 mcg/l, made it next to impossible to advise such a patient at all. The standard textbooks available to physicians, such as the *Cecil Textbook of Medicine*, did not even address fetal exposures.

I gave the obstetrics lecture with one of the high-risk obstetricians in the department. My role was to cover my findings, the levels of mercury in the fish that many people were consuming, the current advisories, and how to advise patients on their diet to obtain omega-3 fatty acids without any significant exposure to methylmercury. My obstetrician colleague spoke first and painstakingly went through the data contained in interim reports from the two major studies of mercury toxicity then being conducted, one in the Seychelles and the other in the Faroe Islands. These two studies were using neuropsychiatric tests to try to determine the lowest level of exposure to methylmercury that affected the fetal brain. They both followed children over time who had been exposed to methylmercury in utero through the mother's fish consumption during pregnancy. The Faroes study found significant exposure-related dysfunctions in the children in most of the neuropsychiatric tests, most pronounced in the domains of language, attention, and memory. The Seychelles study found no adverse effects among subjects with the same exposure levels tested in the Faroes research.[4]

The obstetricians in the audience were concerned about the panic public knowledge of the potential adverse effects of an elevated mercury level would trigger in their pregnant patients. One remarked, "You just can't go and get a mercury level on a pregnant woman and then tell her, oh, by the way you are eating enough mercury that you can potentially cause permanent damage to your baby's brain." Some others agreed and thought broadcast of the dangers of mercury in fish would raise too many questions for already pregnant women and lead to unnecessary concern and abortions. Most physicians in the room agreed that preventive measures were in order, though, and that patients should be advised to avoid consumption of large predatory fish before or during pregnancy. Some later tested their patients and sought my advice. And soon I began to receive calls from my female obstetrician colleagues of reproductive age about their own elevated mercury levels.

In the weeks that followed, various doctors made comments to me, as they tried to make sense of the dilemma. One elder doctor stated, "I have never heard of such a thing—therefore, it couldn't be all that bad." Another said, "You are just trying to scare people." And a third, huffing and puffing as he tried to keep up with me, said smiling, "You ruined my diet."

Not long after the obstetrics talk I was asked to give a grand rounds lecture. Such lectures are a long-standing tradition in medicine. A doctor is invited to give a lecture on a specialty topic of interest to members of the department, including doctors in training, medical students, and anyone else interested in the subject of the lecture. This was my big test: I would be going before my peers in internal medicine in a formal setting. I knew I had to be ready, and I planned the most informative lecture I could.

When I arrived, the atmosphere was friendly and collegial. As I waited to be announced, I scanned the people in the audience, all sitting at tables and facing forward. In age and gender it was a mixed crowd. The moderator, a middle-aged physician who was well established politically at the hospital and seemed always to be in a position where policy decisions were to be made, introduced me, chuckling to himself: "Jane has an unusual interest that has become her religion."

Well, I was not asking anyone to believe in anything, nor was I running for political office, but I proceeded with my lecture. I explained the FDA and EPA advice discrepancies, then the predominant sources of exposure such as inorganic mercury vapor with dental amalgam, methylmercury in fish, and ethylmercury in the vaccine preservative thimerosal, at the time becoming more of a concern in the public eye. I reviewed how organic mercury is excreted mainly in stools, hair, and breast milk but not in urine, whereas inorganic mercury comes out predominantly in the urine, as well as in other bodily fluids. I discussed the nonspecific symptoms I was seeing in my patients compared to the symptoms delineated in the medical texts and told them what tests to order for hair and blood. Analysis of hair and blood, I explained, would give only an estimate of the body load, as certain organs, such as kidney, liver, heart, and brain, take up or hold on to more methylmercury than other parts of the body. I taught them how to estimate a patient's mercury exposure over time using dietary history and a chart of known mercury levels in fish. I then turned to the controversies surrounding chelation treatments that purportedly rid the body of mercury at a faster rate. At the end, an elderly doctor who appeared to have been sleeping for most of the lecture, commented, "I am rather skeptical. We went through this a number of years ago, checking dentists and their personnel and came up with nothing."

I again stressed that inorganic amalgam mercury and methylmercury from fish behaved differently, and it was the latter I was looking into. The politically astute moderator chimed in, "Well, there isn't much here, and there is not enough cause-and-effect data that is significant."

Another physician in the audience opined, "We should not panic the pregnant ladies." At that point, my young female associate, Dr. Nina Simmonds, stood up and declared, "Pregnant women should be allowed to decide their own diet, and the information should be made available to them. Look what happened to the lead issue. The safe level continues to be lowered, and this took a very long time to do because of industry involvement in influencing regulatory agencies."

The moderator countered by asking a doctor whose specialty was the health effects of toxicants found in the workplace for her opinion. Much to my dismay, she said dismissively, "Well, hotdogs don't cause baseball."

I wasn't sure what that meant, but I was left standing in front of my colleagues, some chuckling, some appearing stern, some apparently enlightened, and others concerned. If it were not for the continuing stream of patients coming to my office who were being identified with elevated mercury levels far above what the government said existed in the United States and who seemed to be adversely affected, I might never have opened my mouth about mercury again.

On January 12, 2001, the *20/20* show that featured my patients and the mercury issue finally aired. Senator Patrick Leahy of Vermont came on first. Citing a National Academy of Sciences report released in July of 2000 that reviewed the literature on methylmercury exposure and fish consumption,[5] he announced, "Sixty thousand newborn children may be born with neurological problems that may put them at risk for poor school performance." Later in the program he added, "The good news is we know what the dangers of mercury pollution are; the bad news is our own government is not moving fast enough to do anything about it."

Coal-burning power plants and incinerators were implicated as the current major sources of mercury pollution. The program did not go into detail about the consequence of the mercury being billowed into the air, unfortunately. As explained in the *Mercury Study Report to Congress*, such airborne mercury settles into water bodies, where it is converted to the more dangerous methylmercury by organisms; it then enters the food chain and accumulates as it moves higher in the chain. The longest-lived and most predaceous animals—those that consume the most other contaminated animals—had the highest levels of methylmercury in their bodies. That is why fish like tuna and swordfish are of special concern.[6] When the program turned to mercury in fish, the narrator announced that "three years ago the FDA stopped testing for methylmercury and now requires the fishing industry to police itself."

When asked whether the fishing industry was actually policing itself, Dick Gutting, president of the National Fisheries Institute, countered the implied skepticism by stating, "The average levels are well below the safety limit." The commentator then summarized for the audience Gutting's further comments: "The industry does its own testing, and these tests do not indicate an overall mercury problem [in the fish], although [Gutting] could not site specifics." Arnold Diaz then asked Gutting, "So you have no idea what percentage of the tests that the fisheries are doing are failing [and exceed the FDA action level] on mercury and swordfish." Gutting replied, "That is correct." Diaz then asked, "Then how can you say that there's not a problem?" Gutting replied, "Because if the results are over the limit, the product is not brought into the market."

The industry that was supposed to be policing itself apparently could not or was not willing to provide data to the 20/20 crew. The commentator went on, "But our tests show that some [fish over the 1 mcg/g limit] are ending up in the market. Of forty samples we tested, two of the eighteen tuna tested over the 1 mcg/g limit, two of four shark samples failed, and fourteen of eighteen swordfish failed. Two of the swordfish more than tripled the FDA limit of mercury."

I should reiterate here that for fish to be legally sold on the U.S. commercial market, it cannot contain more than 1 mcg/g of mercury, by the FDA's own standard. That limit was unfortunately not enforceable. Swordfish contained 1.0 mcg/g in mercury on average, which meant that many should be considered unsafe to eat. The industry, though, was not about to test every swordfish that came to the market.

Dr. Jill Stein of Greater Boston Physicians for Social Responsibility was asked to comment on this roulette game consumers were unwittingly playing: "Even a single exposure could potentially harm the fetus at a critical point in brain development," she said.

Diaz commented, "The FDA says it has difficulty taking enforcement action against the industry. So what is the agency doing to protect the public? Well, it's put out an official advisory regarding consumption of high-mercury fish. The problem is many people who need to hear the advice aren't getting it" because about the only place the advisory could be found was on the FDA Web site.

Diaz again: "Both the fishing industry and the FDA say there is no evidence, that most people are [not] eating enough high-mercury fish for it to be a problem. But most people are eating fish for health reasons, like these Californians."

Finally, my patients. Diaz was seen asking them questions, but only a few of them. Most of what was asked during the interviews wound up on the cutting room floor. He then took on the naysayer role himself, claiming that there was no evidence that their elevated mercury levels were dangerous. My only appearance on camera came when the show spliced in my comment for what a pregnant woman should do in regard to fish that could be over the 1 mcg/g limit. I simply stated, "Don't eat it—don't eat that kind of fish." Diaz added, "Dr. Hightower also advises pregnant women to avoid canned tuna, although past FDA tests have shown mercury levels to be far below the limit; they [canned tuna] actually come from a smaller variety of tuna." Unfortunately, he did not make the critical distinction between albacore, or chunk white tuna, which contains three times more mercury than chunk light tuna, which is made up of mostly smaller fish.

In the final comments, Dr. Stein speculated, "The FDA doesn't seem to be paying attention to the science of the last fifteen years." Diaz then added, "For months we have been asking the FDA for an on-camera interview, and they have refused. Interestingly, just this afternoon the FDA announced new guidelines, recommending that pregnant women and young children avoid swordfish and shark altogether."

The other commentator then asked, "Could new warnings do more harm than good?" Dick Gutting responded, "It's awfully easy to scare people with sensational stories, and then they'll stop eating fish, and that's not going to be good for them or their babies." Gutting was ignoring the fact that people who eat a lot of fish—usually high-end consumers—are especially at risk. They would choose the lower-contaminant fish if they had the information. Those who did not like fish would most likely continue not to eat it regardless of the information they received.

Senator Leahy said, "I think it's a no-brainer. Stop the mercury." The commentator summarized his comments by saying, "Senator Leahy says the ultimate solution is tighter restrictions of mercury emissions, but so far he says his proposed legislation has been thwarted by the coal and power plant industries." Leahy was given the show's last word: "We could stop it. We are not stopping it. And until we stop it, we cannot tell our children this is a safe food."[7]

The FDA's new recommendation for that day, I was told later, was not a coincidence. Inconclusive discussions apparently had been going on for a long time, but to those involved in decision making on the issue, my patients and I appeared to simply drop out of the sky. The FDA had left the fishing industry to monitor the mercury in the product the fishing industry was trying to sell. That was scary.

Gutting's comments insinuating that the story of mercury toxicity was sensationalism led some of my patients to feel that they were not taken seriously. They knew how much of their interview was not used and they felt uncomfortable about it. I reassured them that the opposite was true and that they did a good job of bringing awareness to the public about this issue. They stood up for what they thought was right and faced the industry. Theirs was a victory because the FDA was now at least listening.

Someone else was listening, too, apparently. After the 20/20 program, daily canned tuna disappeared from our doctors' dining room at the hospital. Instead, we now began to see a variety of other, more healthful fish served.

Why were the 20/20 people so cautious in their presentation of mercury toxicity? They knew from the experiences of their colleagues that issues involving public health, industry, and government regulation are highly charged. They are played almost like a contact sport. One example was the controversy that had erupted a decade earlier, also over mercury but focused on dental fillings. At that time, the

American Dental Association (ADA), the FDA, the dentists, and the public fought the issue over the airways on the television program *60 Minutes.* Dr. James Adams told me that one of his patients was on the December 16, 1990, program to discuss the issues surrounding mercury/silver tooth fillings. She was suffering from multiple sclerosis, and Dr. Adams thought her amalgams could be contributing to her disease. He therefore removed the fillings, and afterward, she appeared to make a recovery. She went on the program to talk about her experience. Unfortunately, she eventually died of her condition, according to Dr. Adams.

Fillings of this type had been used for almost two hundred years and had sparked controversy in the dental community for just as long. Claims by those interviewed on *60 Minutes* were that the ADA had not sought medical input when addressing the safety of mercury in fillings, that the association was more concerned about lawsuits than the public's health, and that the treatment of anti-amalgam dentists had been ruthless.

By early 1991, the ADA, the FDA, and the *Journal of the American Dental Association* had all released statements to counter the *60 Minutes* program. A report by the U.S. Public Health Service concluded in 1993, "There is scant evidence that the health of the vast majority of people with amalgam is compromised, nor that removing amalgam fillings has a beneficial effect on health. "They also concluded that the possibility that this type of material could pose a health risk could not be ruled out.[8] They therefore recommended a targeted and expanded research program, coordinated by the Public Health Service, to more fully assess the safety of dental restorative materials.[9] The president of the ADA countered many points brought out in the program and charged that "*60 Minutes* chose to present a distorted, inaccurate, biased show that had the effect of frightening thousands of viewers and inappropriately undermining their trust in the dental profession."[10]

I did like the fact that the Public Health Service report also "stressed" and "recommended" that "the manufacturers of all dental restorative materials, including amalgam, be required to disclose the ingredients of those products in the labeling, so that dentists could help patients avoid substances to which they may be allergic."[11] Dr. Adams had many critics, and when, following the above events, he attended a Dental Society meeting of more than 125 dentists, he unfortunately arrived late and sat down at the last remaining chair at a crowded table. All of the dentists at the table got up and stood at the back of the room for the entire meeting, leaving him alone.

Although the 20/20 producers had mentioned that they did not want a controversy to occur as it had with the 60 Minutes program, it seemed odd to me that so little of the patient information was used in the program, and that the focus seemed mostly on the pollution from coal-fired power plants and how that was causing fish to have high methylmercury levels. Important, but my patients were evidence that this mercury was getting to the consumer and having adverse effects. Greater understanding of these human consequences could have lent more urgency to the regulators of mercury pollution and the polluters, and to the FDA, which was supposed to protect the public from harmful levels of exposure.

In the end, the 20/20 program, along with my patients and my prodding, at least encouraged the FDA to put forth a stricter advisory for mercury and fish, one that was long overdue and had evidently been simmering on the policy makers' back burner for some time. It was a small step in the right direction.

CHAPTER 5

A Spoonful of Mercury

I T DIDN'T TAKE ME LONG to recognize that it was usually my senior colleagues who seemed the most vocal and opinionated about the health impact of mercury, regardless of the form it was in. I often heard declarations like, "We used to use mercury all the time. We even put it in wounds to fight infection. There weren't any problems with this." It is difficult to grasp how recently mercury was positively embraced as a therapeutic by many in the medical community and beyond, despite its recognized unfortunate side effects.

Like those in some other professions, many physicians seemed to continue to work in their field for many years after the conventional retirement time. These senior professionals are our eyes of the past. In our institution, this made for an interesting mix of senior wisdom and youthful energy in the small, cramped dining room where we gathered for lunch. My senior colleagues all seemed to remember well the days in the early part of their careers when they and their colleagues routinely prescribed mercurial medicines. Even my eighty-four-year-old father-in-law, who still assisted in surgeries and saw patients in his office, recalled the days of bichloride of mercury and Mercurochrome. The troubling fact, though, when it came to the attitudes of the doctors who prescribed them, is that the old mercurial drugs, vaccines, and salves seldom, if ever, underwent clinical trials that would meet today's standards for assessing either their safety or their effectiveness. Mercury's past, it was clear, was a key to understanding some of the attitudes toward it today.

The agency that eventually became the Food and Drug Administration officially began regulating food and drugs in 1906 with the Federal Food and Drugs Act, often referred to as the Wiley Act. This act made it unlawful for any person to manufacture, sell, or transport adulterated, misbranded, poisonous, or deleterious foods, drugs, medicines, or liquors. The Department of Agriculture and its Bureau of Chemistry enforced the law by testing the products themselves until 1927 when the law enforcement functions were separated from agricultural research. The Food, Drug, and Insecticide Administration was then formed and was renamed the Food and Drug Administration in 1931. The greatest opposition to the 1906 law came from whiskey distillers and patent medicine firms. Their argument was that the federal government had no business policing what people ate, drank, or used for medicine. In any case, little was done to enforce the provisions of the Wiley Act. Though the act allowed for the regulation of a drug's strength, quality, and purity in order to reduce fraudulence, few regulations were put in place, and false therapeutic claims for drugs and adulterated food continued to flourish. When a challenge did arise, a defendant had only to show that he personally believed in his fake remedy to escape prosecution.[1]

In 1938, one hundred people died from a poisonous "elixir of sulfanilamide." This prompted passage of the Federal Food, Drug, and Cosmetic Act, which established higher standards for food and drugs, and stronger federal court injunctions against violators.[2] The act required, among other things, that drug manufacturers provide scientific proof that new products could be safely used before putting them on the market. Proof of fraud was no longer required to stop false claims for drugs. Also, addition of poisonous substances to food was prohibited except where unavoidable or required in production. Despite this effort, the FDA encountered numerous drug manufacturers making false claims about the efficacy of one or another of their new drugs. In response to the tragedy that occurred in Europe, where the sedative thalidomide given to pregnant mothers resulted in the birth of thousands of deformed infants, the Drug Efficacy Amendment of 1962, also known as the Kefauver-Harris Amendment, was made law. This amendment required drug manufacturers to show "proof of efficacy." It also required drug advertising to disclose accurate information about side effects and efficacy of treatments.[3] Unfortunately, many drugs, including those laced with mercury, that had been on the market before 1962, and even before 1938 and 1906, were never subjected to this regulatory system and subsequently escaped being tested. Mercury has deep roots in the medical field, as we'll see. Deep wounds, as well.

The roots of modern chemical therapeutics lie in large part in early alchemical practices among the Arabs, which later spread to Europe and elsewhere. Alchemy was the chemistry of ancient times, and its practitioners ranged widely in mixing agents of all sorts in attempts to turn base metals into a more valuable substance, such as gold, or an antidote to aging. Gold was considered the perfect metal by the alchemists, and it was they who found a way to combine mercury with other substances in order to turn poor-grade gold ores—essentially gold salts—into pure gold. Success in the transmutation of metals was known as the "magnum opus," and it was likened to finding "the philosopher's stone" or the "elixir of life," which would cure all diseases and confer eternal youth. Those who were rumored to know the right mixture of elements to achieve such transmutations were revered in some societies and executed in others.[4]

The earliest written evidence that humans knew how to use mercury to get gold was contained in an edict issued by the Roman emperor Diocletian about AD 290. According to Leonard Goldwater's book *Mercury: A History of Quicksilver*, the edict called for the destruction of all works dealing with alchemy and related subjects. Goldwater wrote, "He [Diocletian] feared that artificially created gold would debase the value of the Roman currency or that makers of precious metals might be able to amass large fortunes with which they could subvert the loyalty of public office and even foment revolts against the ruling power of Rome."[5]

In the centuries that followed, various methods were developed for the extraction of gold and silver using mercury. The "patio" method was commonly used by the Spaniards beginning in the 1500s. It consisted of taking gold or silver ores and crushing them into a powder on a large platform, or *patio*. Depending on the type of ore and the salts that adhered to the metal to be extracted, various other salts and mercury had to be added to the mixture, along with water. Mules were commonly employed to trample this muddy mixture for weeks, to the point that it would literally wear their feet down. After the gold and mercury stuck together, or amalgamated, water was poured over the mixture, washing away the fine particles and nonmetal salts that formed in the process, leaving behind the heavier metal amalgam. The amalgam would then be heated, causing the mercury to evaporate and leaving the precious metal.[6] Many variations of this method have subsequently been employed in the United States and elsewhere.

The Arabs appear to have produced the first writings on the uses of mercury in medicine, animal experimentation, and as a poison for suicide and homicide. Their writings on mercury are thought to date from as early as the AD 700s, but it is still debated when and in what region of the world mercury was actually first employed for medicinal purposes.[7]

The use of mercury for many medical conditions spread throughout the world, even though the efficacy of mercury treatments for a variety of conditions was never proven. By 1495, when the first documented syphilis epidemic arose in Europe, mercury quickly became the treatment ingredient of choice in a variety of different formulations. One mercurial medicine was the "blue pill," or "blue mass," composed of mercury, licorice root, honey, sugar, and confection of dead rose petals, commonly used for hypochondriasis and as a purgative, as well as for syphilis.[8]

Pastes and salves using mercury in the treatment of syphilis and other ailments were first concocted using lard. Later, turpentine of Epirus and the resin of birch were used. Some physicians of the fifteenth and sixteenth centuries used horse fat or bear grease in their salves, along with additives such as bellium, the juice of cedar or myrrh, "male incense," mibium, and burning sulfur. Hieronymus Fracastorius (1478–1553) developed a mercury cure for syphilis that combined mercury with black hellebore, orris root, galbanum, asafetida, oil of mastic, and oil of native sulfur. Fracastorius wrote of his treatments:

> Patients, a truce to the disgust which may be caused by this remedy! For [if] it is disgusting, the disease is still more so. Besides, your cure is at this price. So, without hesitation, spread this mix-

ture on your body and cover with it your entire skin, with the exception of the head and of the precordial region. Then, carefully wrap yourself in wool and tow; then get into bed, load yourself with bed covering and thus await until a sweat bathes your limbs with an impure dew. Ten days in succession renew this treatment, for ten entire days you are to undergo this cruel trial whose beneficial effect will not cause you to wait. As a matter of fact, very soon an infallible presage will announce to you the hour of your freedom. Very soon you will feel the ferments of the disease dissolve themselves in your mouth in a disgusting flow of saliva, and you will see the virus evacuate itself at your feet in rivers of saliva. . . . This treatment being completed, you may then, without fear, recall Bacchus to your table and enjoy in full liberty the generous nectars of Phetia, of Falernum, and of Chios.[9]

Although mercury was used for many years for the treatment of syphilis, there was no proof it ever cured anyone, as most subjects who lived long enough would later go on to have tertiary or late syphilis—hence, the old saying that a night with Venus meant a lifetime with Mercury. On occasion, syphilis was known to spontaneously remit on its own without treatment. The mercurial treatment also caused symptoms that were the same as those of the disease itself, such as shaking tremors, nervousness, hearing loss, delerium, and forgetfulness, as well as abdominal pain, joint pain, and general malaise. "The use of mercury in the treatment of syphilis may have been the most colossal hoax ever perpetrated in the history of a profession which has never been free of hoaxes," as Goldwater put it.[10]

Mercuric chloride (HgCl$_2$), also known as corrosive or sweet sublimate, or bichloride of mercury, was once the most commonly prescribed form of mercurial medicine and antiseptic. Not only did it cause the typical symptoms of mercury poisoning such as nervousness, insomnia, tremor, abdominal pain, salivation, and loose teeth when ingested, it also caused corrosion of the tongue, stomach, and intestines. In 1365, recognizing the hazards of this form of mercury, Sienna, Italy, passed a statute making it illegal to sell corrosive sublimate to any slave, freed or otherwise, or to any servant under age twenty. Sale was further restricted to those well known in the apothecary. Many practitioners continued to embrace mercurials, while others developed a distrust of the substance and felt that mercury taken in any form was poisonous. In 1582, Germany's Augsburg Senate warned apothecaries not to prepare or sell any substances known to be dangerous, including all preparations of mercury.[11]

Calomel, or mercurous chloride (Hg_2Cl_2), also raised concerns through the centuries. Because physicians believed that improper liver function was the cause of many diseases and that mercury stimulated the flow of the liver, calomel was used with indiscretion for a variety of disorders beginning in the late 1500s. It became particularly popular in the United States in the 1800s. In one report comparing Kentucky and New Jersey physicians between 1854 and 1887, mercury ranked second only to opium and morphine in total number of prescriptions written.

Calomel's most noteworthy showdown in the medical establishment came on May 4, 1863, when Surgeon General William A. Hammond (1828–1900) wrote his infamous Circular Number 6. He thought that the Union army was abusing the use of calomel, causing melancholy, exhibited in the form of profuse salivation and "mercurial gangrene"—inflammation of the mouth, tongue, and salivary glands that often led to loosened and lost teeth and fatal infections of the mouth and jaw. In the circular, he ordered calomel to be struck from the supply table. He went on to say, "This is done with the more confidence as modern pathology has proved the impropriety of the use of mercury in very many of those diseases in which it was formerly unfailingly administered."[12]

The army doctors, many of whom Hammond thought were unqualified, were furious. The "regulars" (also referred to as allopaths) thought Hammond had "done great and inexcusable injustice to a noble, humane, scientific, and self-sacrificing profession."[13] They also thought he was caving in to the homeopaths, who thought mercury was toxic in all forms. The American Medical Association (AMA) in 1864 formed a committee just to address the circular and asked some army surgeons their opinions of the issue. The army surgeons claimed they had never seen any cases of mercurialism and that Hammond's circular was an "unwarranted assumption of authority, and a reckless attempt to cut the Gordian knot of intricate pathology by the exercise of official power."[14] Hammond was court-martialed shortly thereafter. In 1878, a Senate hearing concluded that his court-martial was politically motivated and that there had been no dereliction of duty or improper misconduct. He was fully exonerated and restored to the U.S. Army with the rank of brigadier general (retired).[15]

Another medical doctor who did not feel mercurials were living up to the claims of safety and efficacy made for them was British physician Thomas John Graham. Writing in the 1920s, he declared that "the immoderate use of mercury was itself a *cause* of hypochondriasis: Calomel and emetics, when frequently repeated and continued, cannot fail to aggravate and confirm the evil they were intended to cure." (Italics in original.) It was not until after 1926, though, that a steady decline in the use of calomel occurred.[16]

The discovery that organic mercurial compounds could be used as a diuretic (a substance that increases urination) came about in 1919 in Vienna. It was observed by a nurse that after giving the mercurial Novosurol intravenously to a child with congenital syphilis who was suffering heart failure, the patient produced massive quantities of urine. The treating physician then gave the drug to other patients with syphilitic heart disease in heart failure. Gradually, by trial and error, he broadened his on-the-job experimentation to include nonsyphilitic heart failure patients.[17]

Although mercurial diuretics temporarily extended the life of many moribund heart failure patients by forcing the kidneys to rid the body of excess fluid, it also was implicated in some deaths. Some died while the medicine was being infused and the needle was still in their arm. As it was later discovered, mercury can have direct toxic effects on the heart, inducing a malignant rhythm known as ventricular fibrillation. Other causes of death or harm attributed to intravenous mercurial diuretics were acute hemorrhagic colitis, which caused the patient to bleed to death, and grand mal seizures in known epileptics. Because these moribund patients were so affected by their disease, often so exhausted they could not move, or with low oxygen and blood flow in their brains, it would have been difficult to sort out which symptoms were from the failing heart and which were from the mercurial diuretic. Some of the other bothersome effects of the mercurial diuretics were rashes and red skin.

Mercurial diuretics given by mouth fared no better. Like other oral mercurials, such as corrosive sublimate, they caused abdominal distress, diarrhea, nausea, and vomiting in some patients. Why some individuals reacted adversely and others did not was never resolved.[18]

Despite such adverse effects, many of these mercurial agents were still in use in the 1970s. Their eventual abandonment came for at least three reasons: newer and safer agents were being discovered, the FDA was urging drug companies to provide evidence of their safety and efficacy, and the World Health Organization (WHO) in 1972 opined that the use of mercurial pharmaceuticals should be discouraged and suitable alternatives sought.[19]

The average dose of mercury in intravenous diuretic preparations was about 40,000 mcg, while blue mass, which continued to be used to treat syphilis into the early twentieth century, contained about 66,000 mcg. The prescription for these agents often called for multiple doses per day. For example, the oral mercurial diuretic mercurophylline called for a two- to four-day course of one or two tablets three times per day. Under the two-tab, three-times-per-day regimen, one would consume 240,000 mcg of mercury per day. The amount of mercury the body actually absorbed is unknown, but it has been speculated that these were near lethal doses.[20]

In 2006 an elder colleague of mine, Dr. Douglas Pinto, who enjoyed talking about history, declared rather matter-of-factly at the lunch table that the old surgeons "even put it [mercury] in the walls of the old Stanford operating room." Not believing this, I researched further. Our hospital librarians, through luck and keen eyes, found the reference to this historical item of interest. Dr. Pinto had graduated from Stanford University School of Medicine in 1956, and a mention of mercurial walls appeared in its yearbook of 1959. As it was explained in the text, Dr. Levi Cooper Lane (1828–1902), the physician who began the Cooper

Medical College (later Stanford University School of Medicine in San Francisco), believed so strongly in the antiseptic properties of bichloride of mercury that he had it added to the plaster mixture that went onto the walls of not just the operating room but the entire Lane hospital in 1875. The hospital is now at rest in some unfortunate landfill, and in its place is the building where my office is located, at 2100 Webster Street.

Also, at the Lane Hospital of 1875, and the Stanford Hospital, built in 1917, which is still standing next door to my office, many surgeons would wash their hands in bichloride of mercury before surgery. Some of the surgeons were known to pour it on the floor, standing in it with rubber boots while they operated, thinking this would ward away infections, which were a terrifying and deadly complication of their craft. Obviously, Dr. Levi Cooper Lane, Dr. Stanley Stillman, and other founding fathers of the Stanford Medical School were not in agreement with Dr. William Hammond, or perhaps they just never heard about the controversy. The effects on the surgeons and anyone else in the room would be of concern, as the mercury would have been absorbed into their systems through air and skin contact. How long those surgeons exposed themselves in their careers is unknown, as rubber gloves soon replaced this mercurial practice.[21]

As for the mercurous and mercuric chloride used by physicians and surgeons for "sterilizing" their instruments, it was discovered as early as the 1930s that mercury was only *bacteriostatic* to many common bacterial pathogens not *bacteriocidal*. In other words, it did not kill all of the organisms but may have slowed some organisms' growth. Still, it took many years to get physicians to stop their use of mercury and move toward safer and more effective agents for sterilization. With the discovery of the uses for penicillin in 1941, many uses for mercurials began to fade rapidly.[22]

Multiple forms of mercury compounds were also given to infants and children. They were used as laxatives, teething powders, antihelmintics (deworming agents), diaper rash creams, and antiseptics— most notably the organic mercurial antiseptic Mercurochrome. Their use was eventually identified as the cause of a condition known as acrodynia or pink disease. Neurological symptoms ranged from tremor and listlessness to coma and death. The affected infants and children also developed headaches, abdominal pain, rashes, and pink skin. Although this syndrome was described as early as 1890, it took until 1948 to link it to the use of mercurials, after many children either died or were neuropsychiatrically injured for life. After the removal of mercury from children's products, pink disease declined markedly. Of scientific importance was that some children with the same exposure were not noticeably affected, just as with adults, and theories as to why this is the case are still being argued.[23]

Despite FDA regulation, the history of pink disease, Hammond's circular, and the existence of many people who opposed the use of mercurials, they continued to be marketed and available for over-the-counter use in the United States. These very old medicines were essentially grandfathered in as new regulations were passed and, therefore, were never put through proper trials to assess safety and efficacy.

In the 1980s the FDA advisory committee said that mercurials should be assessed for their safety and efficacy, and manufacturers were notified. The FDA therefore reclassified mercurials as new drugs not "generally recognized as safe" (GRAS) and effective. It was not until 1998, however, that the remaining twenty over-the-counter mercurials, including the popular tincture Mercurochrome, the leading household antiseptic for decades, met their demise. According to the *Federal Register*, of seventeen mercury active ingredients available for sale, twelve contained merbromin (this includes Mercurochrome), one contained phenylmercuric nitrate (PMA), and seven contained thimerosal. Mercurochrome itself contained 2,700–5,000 mcg of mercury per milliliter. When the FDA gave its final rule to have these agents removed from over-the-counter use, no challenges were brought by the manufacturers to prove safety or efficacy. These products just quietly disappeared.[24]

I still come across patients who have old Mercurochrome that has been sitting on their shelves for decades. I ask them to bring it to the office so I can get rid of it for them. Here is a medicine of yesteryear that people soaked wounds in and dumped down the sink. Now it has to be handled like toxic waste. (If you have any of it, or any other mercury products, call your local health department, municipal waste authority, or fire department to ask how to dispose of it properly.)

Mercury/silver dental amalgam has been surrounded with claims of adverse health effects from the beginning of its use in 1818. It got its start in the United States when two of the five Crawcour brothers, who were well-known dentists in Europe, brought their special blend of mercury/silver amalgam from London to fill "decaying teeth without the slightest pain, heat, or pressure."[25] They called it Royal Mineral Succedaneum. Unfortunately, the fillings would fall out or crack the teeth, leading to "mercury poisoning" in the patients.[26]

As the Crawcour brothers began to take away patients from other dentists, and the public became angry at the quality of the Crawcours' fillings, the first "amalgam war" ensued from 1841 to 1855. The American Society of Dental Surgeons, founded in 1841, convened to discuss the mercury amalgam problem. Two years later, the society concluded by opinion, but not with scientific methods, that "the use of amalgam constitutes malpractice."[27] The declaration of malpractice for using the mercury/silver amalgams resulted in some dentists being suspended from the practice of dentistry. One anti-amalgam dentist, Dr. J. Payne, was so concerned about the toxic effects of mercury in the mouth that he wanted Congress to pass an act "making it a penitentiary offense to place any poisonous substance in teeth that would injure people."[28] On the opposite side of the amalgam war was Dr. Foster Flagg, who opined in the 1870s that gold was the "worst material" and amalgam an "excellent filling material." This period of time was referred to by the dental community as "the new departure." Homeopathic clinicians weighed in, too, arguing that mercury in amalgams "threw the system out of balance" and "caused derangement of the spleen, stomach, liver, kidneys, nerves, mucous membranes, skin, etc."[29] Ironically, in 2006, a patient brought to me a homeopathic remedy, given to her by her homeopath, that contained "mercurius solubilis."

By 1900, the pro-amalgam view was winning out but still with many objections from some observers in the medical and dental communities. More sophisticated tests allowed scientists to measure the amount of mercury vapor given off by the amalgams, though this, too, became a topic of controversy, as the accuracy of the results was initially questioned. By 1986, the American Dental Association felt so strongly that amalgam did not pose a health hazard to the "nonallergenic patient" that it stated that an amalgam's removal from "nonallergenic" patients for the "alleged purpose of removing toxic substances from the body, when such treatment is performed solely at the recommendation or suggestion of the dentist, was improper and unethical."[30] Over the past two hundred years, then, the dental community had made it a malpractice first to install mercury/silver amalgams and then to take them out.

With the development of better testing methods and machines, it was demonstrated by 2006 that the more amalgams in one's mouth, the more mercury was excreted in one's urine. Exposure from today's mercury/silver amalgam has not been shown to cause a blood level greater than 5 mcg/l, however. Some have speculated that the inorganic mercury vapors are absorbed into the tissues too quickly to be measured in the blood, while others believe the amalgams just don't give off enough mercury to raise the blood level. This information is important if the dose-response relationship of toxicity is being investigated. The problem is that there appears to be a genetic component that makes some people more sensitive than others to low exposures of many substances. Bee stings provide a good example. Although it takes about 1,100 bee stings to inject enough venom to kill the average 132-pound person, about one in a thousand humans die from a single sting. In the latter scenario, it is not the toxicology at play, but the body's genetically produced reaction to the toxicant.

Recently, the development of what's called the MELISA (memory lymphocyte immunostimulation assay) test has enabled patients to find out what metals the type of white blood cells known as lymphocytes are reacting to. This type of lymphocyte reaction the MELISA test is detecting is called a type IV allergy and is slow and chronic, unlike the immediate type I anaphylaxis seen with bee stings. The metals found in dental amalgams that are most commonly associated with the type IV allergy are nickel, aluminum, beryllium, copper, indium, inorganic mercury, methylmercury, palladium, silver, and tin. In one study involving

250 patients, the five most common metals that people's lymphocytes reacted to were nickel (73%), titanium (42%), cadmium (18%), gold (17%), and palladium (13%). In 2003, results of the largest MELISA study to date were published. It involved testing more than three thousand patients who complained of various nonspecific symptoms resembling those of chronic fatigue, and who also had a history of intolerance to metals. Nickel was found to be the most common sensitizer, followed by inorganic mercury, gold, cadmium, and palladium. Replacement of amalgam and other dental metals resulted in health improvement for the majority of patients with this type of allergy. Follow-up MELISA tests showed that the severity of those patients' lymphocyte reactivity had also subsided.[31]

One can begin to conclude that for some individuals, it is not the accumulation and high doses of mercury or another metal that are causing the adverse effects, but instead small doses that are registering in their highly sensitive lymphocytes. Also, such individuals may be reacting to the other metals in the amalgam. Perhaps for some people, titanium should be taken out of toothpaste and chewing gum. Regardless, these types of tests are important to shed light on how we may react adversely to some of the many substances we are exposed to in our daily lives.

By the first years of the twenty-first century, the amalgam issue in the United States has not been completely resolved. With the information provided by MELISA; research on protein carriers for metals; and new understanding of the variations among individuals in detoxification pathways, genetic predispositions, and the synergistic properties among metals and chemicals people are exposed to, perhaps we will find useful answers to many such questions in the near future. In the meantime, because so many scientific papers indicate that mercury/silver amalgam can lead to adverse health effects in some individuals, some countries, including Germany and Sweden, have been phasing out the use of metals in restorative dental materials. As better dental restorative materials continue to be developed, the mercury/silver amalgam controversy may eventually become moot. Regardless, in the United States in 2006, the FDA still stated that these types of amalgams were safe, while the FDA's own advisory committees continued to advise otherwise.

While supporters of mercury dental amalgam are trying to maintain its place in the health care industry, supporters of another mercury dinosaur, the "preservative" thimerosal, otherwise known as Merthiolate, are trying to hold on to its position. Thimerosal, first patented and used in commerce by Eli Lilly and Company in 1928, contains ethylmercury. In its patent, Lilly and Co. claimed that thimerosal was useful in antisepsis and treatment of nose and throat infections.[32] Lilly scientists Jamieson and Powell and others set out to show thimerosal's usefulness in many applications. They claimed in scientific journals that it had excellent wound healing capacity due to its antiseptic properties; preservative success in human tissues; preservative properties in vaccines, especially where multiple doses are drawn; and germicidal effect.[33] Later studies showed these claims to be inaccurate, as the mercurials, including thimerosal and bichloride of mercury, did not kill many of the organisms tested or preserve sterility in surgical instruments or biological products, tissues for transplant and vaccines included. Merthiolate/thimerosal at one time was the most popular medium for storing cartilage in clinical use—until it was discovered that it killed the cartilage cells, making the cartilage nonviable. Thimerosal did, however, have some bacteriostatic properties. In other words, as explained earlier, although it did not kill many bacteria, it might slow the action down of some.[34]

Today's flavor of the debate on the safety of thimerosal can be captured by looking at the research and conclusions of two different teams of scientists. The first team, led by Michael Pichichero of the University of Rochester, published a paper in the British medical journal the *Lancet* in 2002.The authors looked into the mercury concentrations and metabolism of infants receiving vaccines containing thimerosal. Forty infants six months of age and younger were given diptheria–tetanus–acellular pertussis vaccine (DTaP) and hepatitis vaccine, and some infants were also given haemophilus influenza type B vaccine. Total mercury levels were measured three and twenty-eight days after the vaccine was given. The authors concluded, "The administration of

vaccines containing thimerosal does not seem to raise blood concentrations of mercury above safe levels." They went on to say, that the results
of their study "showed that amounts of mercury in the blood of infants
receiving vaccines formulated with thimerosal were well below concentrations potentially associated with toxic effects."[35]

It would have been better if the authors had followed the infants for
a longer period of time, even through their formative years, to see if any
effects truly did not appear. There were few data on the differences
between methylmercury and ethylmercury, they said, and how infants
metabolized ethylmercury was unknown, but they used the risk assessments from methylmercury literature for their interpretation, anyway.
There also was no discussion of possible differences between the
effects of a one-time large dose of three thimerosalized vaccines and
the effects of a lower chronic dose, which could occur from consuming methylmercury in food. Currently, it is unknown how much mercury given to a developing brain—and at what stage of development
—will lead to harmful effects. There didn't seem to be adequate data in
the study to back up the safety claims made by the Rochester group.
In the paper, the authors declared no conflicts of interest, but after
further research into lead author Dr. Pichichero's publications and
Web site, I discovered that he was actually a major vaccine developer
and researcher. As such, he has received grants and honoraria from,
and has served as a consultant for, major vaccine manufacturers,
including Eli Lilly. He has done a considerable amount of research in
developing vaccines that do and do not contain mercury as a preservative.[36] In 2008, in the journal *Pediatrics*, another paper led by
Pichichero was published that again addressed thimerosal in vaccines.
This time it was concluded that in light of the short half-life of ethylmercury, a new risk assessment of exposure needs to be conducted, as
the fate of mercury after it leaves the infant's blood and is dispersed
through its body before elimination is unknown.[37] In other words,
although the mercury left the *blood* quickly, the scientists recognized
this time that mercury may not leave the *body* quickly without going
into other organs first.

Vaccines truly have saved lives, and Dr. Pichichero's work is needed, but every scientist in publications should reveal conflicts of interest and uphold the rules of disclosure. After all, the *Lancet* does have this policy in their rules for authors. So does the journal *Pediatrics*. No financial conflicts were identified by the authors in that paper either. Readers should be allowed to decide for themselves whether a conflict may have contributed to how the researcher "interpreted" the data.

The second team is led by two men by the name of Mark and David Geier. They have been searching the Centers for Disease Control (CDC) databases to see whether there was increased reported incidence of neurodevelopmental disorders and heart disease in children receiving thimerosalized versus nonthimerosalized DTaP vaccines. They published some of their most often cited works in 2003. They observed "statistically significant increases in the incidence rate of neurodevelopmental disorders after the thimerosal-containing DTaP in comparison with thimerosal-free DTaP." The Geier and Geier papers led to rather rigorous discussions, and they received criticism on every aspect of their research imaginable, from the way they gathered the data to their interpretation of the data.[38]

The preservative effectiveness of ethylmercury against bacteria that can be introduced by multiple needle insertions to a multidose vial of vaccine is questionable. But what we now know is that mercury stimulates lymphocytes, which in turn are involved in the production of antibodies. The vaccine is given in order to increase antibodies to a specific antigen (viral protein). Higher antibody production in response to the vaccine is thought to mean that the vaccine is more effective.

Many vaccine manufacturers are now using aluminum to enhance the antibody response (that is, as an adjuvant), and as of 2005, aluminum was the only FDA-approved metal adjuvant. One could then ask whether thimerosal functions as an adjuvant more than as an antiseptic. To claim it as an adjuvant, though, the manufacturers would have to prove safety and efficacy. It was easier just to stick to the claim that it was an antiseptic, as that notion had been grandfathered in. Regardless, out of concern about the amount of mercury in vaccines, along with the increased number of vaccines given to infants, in 1999 the FDA requested manufacturers to reduce the amount of thimerosal in—or eliminate thimerosal from—vaccines and to test the products again for sterility, potency, stability, and immunogenicity (effectiveness). Since then, thimerosal-free vaccines have been made available. Since the new adjuvant, aluminum, is widespread in the food we eat and appears to be less toxic than mercury, you can expect it to be the most commonly used adjuvant for at least the near future. Only time will tell whether we have made the right choice, and many interested parties are watching closely this time.[39]

Perhaps the most egregious claim for Merthiolate, or thimerosal, in its early history was that it cured the common cold. In a 1935 paper, I noticed that the decongestant ephedrine was in the mix for the remedy, but Merthiolate got the credit. No control group was used. This "cure" was soon discredited by a subsequent study in which a control population was used and ephedrine was not given to the study subjects. [40]

A major concern discussed recently in the media is whether mercury could cause autism. Autism spectrum disorders (ASDs) are a group of childhood developmental disorders characterized by impaired social interaction and communication, and by repetitive or stereotypical behavior. The prevalence of ASD in developed countries is estimated to be at least sixty per ten thousand births. The current consensus among scientists is that it is heritable but influenced by environmental triggers. The diagnosis of ASD has been the most elusive diagnosis in children of our time. Different genes have been proposed as the cause of different types of autism. Factors currently being researched include infectious causes; immune dysfunction; abnormalities in neurotransmitters; hormone disturbances or exposures; prescription drugs; illicit drugs; alcohol; smoking; and environmental toxicants, including mercury and air pollutants. So far, factors that have been most consistently associated with autism are uterine bleeding in pregnancy, caesarian section, low birth weight, preterm delivery, and low Apgar score.[41]

The debate continues on whether mercury/thimerosal, methylmercury in fish, or inorganic mercury in amalgams has caused adverse development outcomes such as autism and learning disorders in some children. It is important that all types of mercury exposures be taken into consideration, as well as other numerous exposures children are being subjected to. Genetics does seem to be playing a major role when it comes to the amount of mercury it takes to cause adverse effects, and the types of effects expressed in a given individual. Since none of us knows whether we possess the protective genes or the susceptible ones, precaution is in order for all. Methylmercury can penetrate every cell in the body. It interferes with a myriad of body pathways and stops cell division and thus cell generation by interfering with the apparatus (microtubules) that divides the cell. The longer and more intense the exposure, the higher chance it has of causing harm.

For the last spoonful of mercury in medical history, the long alliance the fishing industry has had with the health care and pharmaceutical industries—especially with cod liver oil and therapeutics deserves mention, as the fishing industry often counters evidence of mercury's harm with fish oil's benefit. Medicinal properties of fish oil have been known as far back as Hippocrates (460–370 BC). Fish oil became more documented in the 1800s as a treatment for rheumatism, osteomalacia (softening of bones), rickets, scrofula (tuberculosis of the neck), general tuberculosis, gout, and infections. As the demand for the oil increased, impurities and fraud plagued the industry, as many proprietors tried to substitute other oils for cod liver oil. In the 1920s it was discovered that vitamins A and D, rich in cod liver oil, were the therapeutic agents that could account for some of the good effects. By the 1930s, at the request of the American Medical Association and the U.S. Public Health Service, vitamin D was added to milk, and in the 1940s vitamin A was added.[42] The use of cod liver oil then waned, but it was still in use for those who could not drink milk or get adequate sunshine and therefore were at risk for vitamin deficiency. In the 1970s, cod liver oil made a comeback when its other healthful components—the omega-3 fatty acids, which can be found in fish in general—were discovered. (The milk industry continues to be a strong competitor as a source of similar benefits. I recently noticed that some brands of milk have now added omega-3 fatty acids from nonfish sources.)

The fishing industry has had great success in having its products promoted as healthful and even curative by the medical establishment.

But within fish protein lie varying levels of mercury. This contaminant can be distilled out of the commercial oil preparations, but it cannot be taken out of the fish one consumes. And it's to the checkered history of mercury's darker side that we now turn.

CHAPTER 6

Making Money with a Menace

THAT MERCURY EXPOSURE sometimes has devastating effects on humans has been recognized for centuries. Among the groups most likely to suffer have been mercury miners, goldsmiths, tinsmiths, and mirror makers, who often developed symptoms from mercury vapor exposure in their occupations. Some of the centuries-old texts described their symptoms in detail, using the colorful yet descriptive medical terms of their era. Workers exposed to mercury, it was reported, developed vertigo (dizziness), asthma, paralysis, palsy of the neck and hands, loss of teeth, uncertain gait, and scelotyrbe (an old term for Parkinson's). According to the founder of occupational and industrial medicine, physician Bernardino Ramazzini (1633–1714), "Very few [mercury-exposed workers] reached old age, and it was also said that even if they did not die young, their health was so terribly undermined that they prayed for death."[1]

The history of workers in the hat-making industry is the most cited incidence of mercury poisoning and became a sad lesson in the annals of occupational health. The hat-making industry used mercury nitrate in the nineteenth and early twentieth centuries to make fur pelts more soft and pliable. Although the first clinical description of "mercurialism" in hatters was published in the transactions of the Medical Society in New Jersey in 1860, it was not until 1937 that the U.S. Public Health Service, with the cooperation of the hatters' union, studied and reported on affected workers, 40 percent of whom were women and more than 75 percent of whom were foreign born. The exposed workers complained of "the shakes"; tremor; gastrointestinal disturbances; sore mouth; psychic disturbances such as irritability, timidity, irascibility, and difficulty in getting along with people; headaches; drowsiness;

insomnia; and weakness. Extensive mercury absorption over long periods of time was associated with elevated risk in cardiovascular disturbances of the "hypertensive type."[2]

In May 1951 the one-hundredth anniversary of the formation of the
hatters' union was celebrated in Danbury, Connecticut, where one of
the largest hat-making industries once thrived. Luckily, a descendant of
a hatter kept the union document that reported this event and kindly
sent a copy to me. In it, one worker recalled, "So much steam, you
didn't only want to wear a rubber apron in front of you, but also over
your head; there wasn't any ceiling; the steam rising to the rafters, con-
densed and came down like rain." The report went on: "Unknown to
the workers it was a rain of death from the fumes of nitrate of mercury."
Another worker declared, "If a worker knew he was getting the shakes,
he would try to hide it. . . . I suspect I had it too, but I wouldn't go to
the doctor. If a worker claimed compensation, he got on the blacklist of
the manufacturers—he couldn't get another job unless he'd sign a
waiver against future claims."[3]

Despite years of accumulated evidence, it was not until 1941 that
mercury was finally removed from the process of making hats. Recent
soil samples showed high mercury levels where much of the Danbury
hat industry was located, and the area was declared an EPA Superfund
cleanup site.[4] It was the hatting industry that gave us the terms "Danbury shakes" and "mad as a hatter," and it then left us with a mess to
clean up.

Occupations from tinsmithing to mirror making often detailed using
mercury routinely, despite the evident harm to workers. Mercury's most
unholy alliance, though, was undoubtedly with gold. Drawing the gold
content from rocks seemed to most people a mystical feat. The salts
and other minerals that were used in the process were even thought to
have medicinal value. The gold itself became desirable for many reasons and quickly became a form of currency.

The quest for gold is most likely what led initially to massive mining
for mercury, or, as the ore was once known, cinnabar. The largest of the
early mercury mines was located in Spain, at Almaden, whose name is
thought to be derived from the Arab term *al-madin*, or "the mine."

Mercury mines were known to be operating in Spain as early as the fourth century BC, but for what purpose mercury was extracted in those early years is still unclear. Arabs, Spanish monarchies, Romans, Christian religious orders, military groups, and private industry have all had their hand in the fight for control of the mines over many centuries.[5]

King Ferdinand V and Queen Isabella saw amassing gold as a critical means of building Spain into a wealthy and powerful Christian empire. On March 31, 1492, they encouraged Arabs to leave the country and ordered Jews out of Spain by July 31, 1492. The last Jews left August 2. On August 3, Christopher Columbus set sail in search of gold, land, and subjects for Christian conversion and colonization. Some have speculated that the date was no accident, as he may have needed to leave then with the Jews that were to serve on his ship. In his letter of proposal to the king before his departure, he had vowed that the colonists would be forbidden to seek gold without a license and would be required to register all gold that they found. In addition, he wrote, "One per centum of all the gold that may be found shall be set aside for building churches and adorning the same, and for the support of the priests or friars belonging to them." Columbus even proposed that the gold be split fifty-fifty with the king of Spain and said, "In the eagerness to get gold, everyone will wish, naturally, to engage in its search in preference to any other employment."[6]

Columbus was the first to take mercury to the New World, on his second voyage, in 1494, as he expected to find gold then in the Antilles. The Spanish colonists did not transport large quantities of mercury until the mid-sixteenth century, though, when it was imported to Mexico from Almaden and Iridia in the Austrian Alps for the amalgamation of silver from ore using the patio process in which mercury was added to ore crushed on a platform.[7]

When the Spaniards found cinnabar in Huancavelica, Peru, in 1563, the Spanish crown established a monopoly on all production, shipment, and sale of the metal. It instituted a forced-labor system, called the mita system, in which all Indians were obligated to work in the mercury mines for a period of six months every two to three years.

Juan de Solórzano Pereira, who was in charge of the Huancavelica mines from 1616 to 1619, wrote in 1648, "Sooner or later even the strongest *mitayos* [workers] succumbed to mercury poisoning." He went on to say that he had never known one who had survived this condition for more than four years.[8] Another historian writing about the mitayos noted that the use of coca leaf was "an indispensable source of sustenance during Andean labor."[9] This fact will come to play a role, we'll see, in a subsequent study of the effects of mercury exposure.

In 1558, Spanish ships began to transport liquid mercury (quicksilver) by the ton from Almaden and Huancavelica to Potosi, Bolivia, and Vera Cruz, Mexico, for mining.[10] Unfortunately, many of the ships did not reach their destination. It has been estimated that in the span of 350 years, Spain annually lost about ten ships, some of them undoubtedly carrying significant amounts of mercury, to hurricanes, pirates, or other catastrophes.[11] To extract gold and silver in quantity, massive amounts of mercury were needed. More than fifty thousand tons of quicksilver were likely brought to Vera Cruz alone, and only now are its impacts beginning to be investigated in parts of Mexico. In some locally grown corn in El Pedernalillo, mercury from earlier mining activities was measured at one hundred parts per million (mcg/g), according to a 2002 report.[12]

The largest known loss of mercury-laden vessels was that of the *Nuestra Señora de Guadalupe* and the *Conde de Tolosa* in 1724.[13] The silver master Don Francisco Barrero y Peláez had planned for the mercury shipment, enough for a year's extraction, to begin its journey from Cádiz in July, arriving in Vera Cruz by September. The *Nuestra Señora de Guadalupe* held 250 tons of quicksilver and the *Conde de Tolosa* held 150 tons. The two ships, their cargo, 144 cannons, and twelve hundred colonists and crew set sail in July as planned, and all went well until August 23, when the winds began to pick up as the travelers drew near Hispaniola. The big galleons were thrown off course and were separated, each alone to fight the wind and seas when the hurricane struck. The cannons on board broke loose and were tossed about the decks, as mountains of water ripped everything topside, including the masts. The *Guadalupe* drove deep into a sandbar in Samana Bay, where the passengers were able to ride out the next day's storm and many were able then to reach shore.[14] The *Tolosa* made it to the mouth of Samana Bay but broke apart on a coral reef. Of the six hundred people aboard, only eight men managed to climb the rigging and ride out the storm. Seven would survive to tell their story, after collecting water to drink in the wind-torn sails, eating any edible floating cargo, and watching the sharks devour the dead below.

Ships ordered from Santo Domingo to recover the precious cargo found the men thirty-two days later. Divers made many attempts at recovery of the cargo, diving with only their one breath in shark-infested waters. The divers to the *Guadalupe* were unable to gain access to the mercury because heavy ship fittings blocked entry to the cargo hold; the heavy timbers of the *Tolosa* had swelled in the salty sea, sealing the cargo door beyond the efforts of the divers. For two and a half centuries, the glass jars that contained the quicksilver continued to break with each storm, resulting in the sinking of nearly all of the mercury to the middle of the bay.[15]

One treasure diver, reporting on the site to his investors, wrote, "Large quantities of free flowing mercury are scattered throughout the wreck sites, and we expect to find large quantities of mercury enclosed in olive jars that remain buried in the sand. It is possible that 1,000,000 lbs. of mercury may be recovered."[16] Unfortunately, they were not able salvage the mercury at the time, and it lies there along with mercury that has made its way from land in the process of gold mining. Treasure divers and their lawyers recently told me that they could remove more of the mercury off the ships—with better resources and money, that is. However, with the reduction of mercury use in industry, the cost to treasure divers to salvage it exceeds its current value.

Many reports of mercury contamination of the fish in the seas of the Americas, especially near the eastern shores, say only that the mercury came from mining as it was transported to lakes and streams. In light of the shipwrecks now known of, perhaps, we will also look at the mercury that was accidentally dumped directly on the ocean floor before it ever got to a small stream in the hills for gold and silver processing. The people of Peru, the Amazon, Colombia, and the Caribbean have all paid the price for mercury pollution, as the mercury made its way to fish and then humans.[17]

Gold mining using mercury has been a major source of environmental contamination nationwide in the United States, especially in states such as California, Nevada, Idaho, and Colorado. Although my family has held mining claims for more than one hundred years, I do not currently know whether any family members used mercury while mining. But my grandfather, born in 1885, was the son of a gold miner, and I remember as a young girl hearing his stories of watching as a boy how the Chinese workers would be "working the sluice boxes." Those boxes would run mercury and sediment together for an amalgamation process to collect gold. Just as with the hatting industry, having foreign, uneducated, or desperate peoples conduct the dangerous jobs seemed to be commonplace at that time; this can still be seen in other industries today. Because of using mercury in the mining process, many lakes, streams, and rivers have been severely contaminated with mercury. The EPA, the United States Geological Survey (USGS), the Department of Fish and Game, the Public Health Department, and environmentalists continue to monitor all aspects of this destructive practice that occurred for many years and poisoned the streams, the fish and waterfowl we eat, and other animals that rely on the waterways for their survival.

Our waterways have also been subject to mercury pollution from paper and pulp mills and from chlor-alkali, cement-making, and other plants. These industries, as we will see, have played a major role in mercury pollution history. Other indirect sources of mercury pollution in our waterways include hospital incinerators, crematoria, and coal-burning power plants that emit various forms of mercury into the air from their stacks. The mercury then falls onto the land and water and is converted to methylmercury, which accumulates as it makes its way through the food chain.

All this pollution has resulted in fish consumption advisories for most water bodies in the United States. Freshwater fish are mostly under the jurisdiction of the EPA and are less commonly sold commercially. The extent of mercury and other contaminants such as polychlorinated biphenyls (PCBs), cadmium, and various pesticides found in freshwater fish varies from one water body to the next; therefore, each state has its own set of advisories. Some of the freshwater fish that can test high in mercury include largemouth and smallmouth bass, yellow perch, walleye, pickerel, northern pike, rock bass, trout, bluegill, and bullhead.[18] As of this writing, many fish obtained through sport fishing, or the commercial market, have yet to undergo adequate testing for contaminants.

One of the chemical industries most notorious for mercury pollution has been the chlor-alkali manufacturing industry, which produces chlorine, a chemical that is widely used in swimming pools, common household bleach, and the plastics industry. While fifty-three plants in the United States had changed to a nonmercury system by 2000, nine plants in eight states (Alabama, Delaware, Georgia, Louisiana, Ohio, Tennessee, West Virginia, and Wisconsin) still had not. One of the nine has agreed to convert to a mercury-free system, while another announced plans for closure. Mercury emitted from these plants into air and water becomes methylmercury and bioaccumulates in the surrounding fish and other wildlife. In recent years, these plants were required to report their mercury emissions and off-site disposals each year. In 2003, an EPA report in the *Federal Register* announced that the annual mercury emission figures for these nine plants amounted collectively to about eight tons, and another six tons were attributed to "fugitive emission." In 2000, a problem arose when the nine mercury-based chlorine plants reported that seventy-nine tons of mercury had been consumed during the manufacturing process, but only fourteen tons were reported released. This left sixty-five tons unaccounted for in that year. The EPA responded to this discrepancy by saying, "The fate of all the mercury consumed at mercury-cell chlor-alkali plants remains somewhat of an enigma." The industry claimed that the remainder of the mercury was contained on site within the manufacturing infrastructure and processing equipment. Regardless, the EPA has sought to limit mercury emissions from these plants under the provisions of the Clean Air Act. In 2006, the American Medical Association (AMA), recognizing that not enough progress had been made toward reduction of mercury from these types of plants, urged state governments to protect their citizens from mercury emissions and encouraged the reduction in mercury use in manufacturing whenever possible.[19]

The AMA certainly has made progress in its opinion about mercury since 1864 and the Hammond-versus-the-army-surgeons' calomel war. I was surprised, though, that in this day and age, there were still industries directly dumping any contaminant into the ground, air, or water. Perhaps the term "contaminant" needs to be redefined. Or perhaps they are having trouble with the terms "dumping" and "emissions."

Perhaps the managers and owners of these plants did not know about, had forgotten, or chose to ignore the plight of the people of Minamata, Japan. It was in that small factory town dominated by the Chisso Corporation that mercury pollution took a tremendous toll and became known around the world, in no small part because of the documentary work of the photojournalists and investigative reporters W. Eugene and Aileen Smith.[20]

Formed in 1907, the Chisso Corporation began as a carbide and fertilizer company. Because the company recognized that dumping chemicals into the bay might be harming the fish supply, in 1925 it began paying the local fishermen a small "indemnity" for the damage they were causing. In 1932, Chisso began to produce acetaldehyde, a component used in the manufacturing of plastics, drugs, perfumes, and photographic chemicals, and by the 1950s it had become one of the largest producers of acetaldehyde in the world. Unfortunately, it used mercury as a catalyst in the process.

In 1956, a "strange disease" became evident and was soon termed "Minamata disease." One day a five-year-old girl was brought to the Chisso company hospital suffering from symptoms of severe brain damage, as she could not talk or walk and was delirious. Several days later, her two-year-old sister was brought to the hospital with the same symptoms. The Smiths interviewed the neighbors of these two little girls, who described them as the "brightest, most vibrant, cutest kids you could imagine" before they were stricken with the illness. Many others followed, and thoughts that the disease was contagious brought fear to the neighboring people.

Then something else unusual was noticed in the neighborhood:

After people's cats began walking in an uncoordinated way and acting erratically, sometimes jumping into the bay, they all disappeared. A Chisso hospital doctor, Hajimé Hosokawa, began an investigation of what lay behind the mysterious illness. He concluded that the malady was not contagious and that the outbreak could be traced to the fish diets of both the people and the cats. After some investigators began claiming that Chisso was pouring nearly sixty kinds of poison into the bay, the factory managers and the residents both began digging in their heels. Chisso then decided to dump its wastewater into the Minamata River delta on the other side of town instead of into the bay. Within a few months, the disease had followed. In 1959, a group from Kumamoto University reported that organic mercury was the cause of Minamata disease. Despite this, confusion persisted. "Chisso shadow-boxed and, I suspect, paid experts to refute every report and every derogatory theory," the Smiths write.

Meanwhile, Dr. Hosokawa, Chisso's investigator, continued giving cats multiple substances to see what might cause the symptoms of Minamata disease. Then he simply gave effluent waste from the acetaldehyde waste pipe to cat number 400. Later, the cat convulsed, salivated, and began to behave in the erratic way of the Minamata-diseased cats. As the Smiths write, "[Hosokawa] was allegedly 'forbidden' more of the effluent and was 'taken off' of the experiments," and Chisso allegedly "hid" Hosokawa's "proof." Chisso then began negotiations with the patients, and fishermen stormed the factory demanding further indemnity. For decades thereafter, a protracted back-and-forth battle among the factory, the Japanese government, the "experts," and the people ensued. At one point, Eugene Smith was severely beaten by a mob of workers at the Chisso plant as he tried to observe and report on what was happening in the plant in regard to this disastrous poisoning. He nearly lost his life and suffered permanent blindness and chronic headaches. He died six years later. His wife, Aileen, now lives in Japan and still is active in her mission to protect the public from pollution.[21]

Unfortunately, the Chisso Corporation did not stop its pollution and admit to its practices in a timely fashion. As a result of its denials, other companies continued to pollute as well. In 1966, the Showa Denko factory was discovered to be dumping chemical waste into the Agano River, affecting at least five hundred people in the community of Niigata forty miles downstream with methylmercury poisoning. In 1967 the victims brought suit against the company for what the lawyers termed Niigata-Minamata disease. "Awkward as it sounds," they said, "we want everyone who hears of this to realize that it isn't just Niigata's little local problem."[22] Ten years later, as we'll see, this Niigata incident became more important, as information on two of its victims was used by the World Health Organization to discern how much methylmercury in methylmercury-contaminated fish it took to cause harm.

The Chisso Corporation refused to accept the blame or responsibility for years, arguing that the people were not affected by effluent from its plant. Massive protests took place in Japan periodically, as more people kept coming forward with health claims and symptoms that would be declared as "lesser Minamata" in the years that followed.

In 1974, the Japanese government put together a list of criteria for Minamata disease that would be used to determine who was eligible for monetary compensation. According to environmental epidemiology professor Toshihide Tsuda of Okayama University, the Japanese government has yet to explain the scientific basis of the criteria. When Dr. Tsuda asked how the criteria were derived, the government told him, "The documentation existed, but we lost it." In 1996, the Japanese government finally agreed to readdress the complaints of the victims and reconsider the symptoms that would qualify for Minamata disease. By March 1997, more than seventeen thousand people had applied for monetary relief and medical subsidies. According to Dr. Tsuda's calculations, however, even in 2008 some people with more than a 99 percent medical probability of having Minamata disease are not recognized under the present system.[23]

Aileen and Eugene Smith suspected that Chisso or the government "paid experts to refute every report and every derogatory theory." In the prologue to their book, Eugene seems perturbed that even someone at a 1970 mercury conference at the University of Rochester tried to discourage him from going to Japan to investigate the mercury situation there, saying, "Why bother going when the incident is over?"[24]

As for the "lesser" symptoms of mercury, large epidemiologic studies conducted in Japan in the last eight years have revealed that a variety of symptoms—such as fatigue, muscle and joint pain, inability to organize one's thoughts, incoordination, memory loss, insomnia, dizziness, tremor, and numbness—occur with statistical significance at mercury levels lower than 50 mcg/l. More recent papers show that subjective complaints have occurred more commonly in the Minamata pollution area than among those living in other areas, but mercury levels of the study subjects were unfortunately not disclosed. Despite the recent scientific papers broadening the clinical depiction of Minamata disease, it appears that the government of Japan still does not recognize some of these symptoms as part of the Minamata diagnostic criteria and adheres to its 1974 algorithm.[25]

The Chisso Corporation did finally pay over $86 million in compensation and was ordered to clean up its contamination. But this judgment occurred in 2004, decades after the initial cases of mercury poisoning were reported.[26] Japan's supreme court ruled that the state was responsible for the spread of Minamata disease after January 1960. Justice Kitagawa said, "As of November 1959, the defendants would have known that there were scores of Minamata disease sufferers and that many of them had died," according to a *Japan Times* article in October 2004. He went on to say, "It was very irrational and illegal for the central government and Kumamoto Prefecture, based on existing laws and regulations at the time, to not clamp restrictions on the wastewater after January 1960."[27] More than seventeen hundred people were estimated to have been killed by the disease and many more harmed. According to news accounts at the time, the environment minister Yuriko Koike made a deep bow to the plaintiffs in a meeting after the verdict and said, "The government will tell about the lessons learned here for generations to come."[28] Perhaps we are still learning our lessons, as compensation to hundreds of victims who should have qualified for compensation has yet to come.

Although many industries have stopped or markedly reduced their mercury emissions in recent years, coal-burning power plants remain a major source of mercury emissions. Recent estimates of annual total global mercury emissions from all sources—both natural and human-generated—range from roughly 4,400 to 7,500 tons per year. Human-caused U.S. mercury emissions are estimated to account for roughly 3 percent of the global total, and U.S. coal-fired power plants are estimated to account for about 1 percent.[29] Because I was concentrating on patients exposed to mercury from fish consumption, I at first didn't realize the role of the energy industry in the mercury policy and regulatory process. Opposition to the notion that people in the United States could consume enough mercury to do them harm just by eating commercial fish, as we'll see in later chapters, was not coming from the fishing industry alone.

Methylmercury is considered more hazardous than most chemicals in four out of four ranking systems. It is also ranked as one of the most hazardous compounds (worst 10%) to ecosystems and human health.[30] Therefore, there has never been a published report of deliberately giving methylmercury to humans to identify the full spectrum of side effects. It would be considered unethical by most if not all institutional review boards. Despite this, even today there exist religious practices in which people apparently have little concern about wearing quicksilver in containers around their neck, rubbing it in their hair, or injecting it into their skin to ward off evil spirits—while other individuals are trying to rid their body of every trace or form of mercury.[31]

Through the centuries, some of the most mercury-exposed people have been the industrial workers and miners themselves and the fishermen who ate the fish tainted with the mercury pollution of years past. Many animals have also been adversely affected by mercury that polluted their habitats and subsequently their bodies. To have a better understanding of the full spectrum of mercury effects, we must rely on epidemiologic studies of populations already exposed. Finding the population that would give us the best and most reliable information has proven challenging. In Minamata and Niigata, mercury levels unfortunately in the victims were not obtained at the time of exposure, and levels drawn later were deemed inaccurate.

Miners, fishermen, and animals have become study subjects of special interest today, but trying to identify correlations of subjective complaints and subtle neurologic changes with methylmercury can be tedious. Study subjects may also have a vested interest in the outcome of such research. They may be reluctant to come forward or give full disclosure of any illnesses because of the possibility of losing their jobs for having done so or suffering financial loss or other repercussions in their business from the unfavorable outcome of a study. Animals, on the other hand, may develop some obvious physical effects with significant exposure, but subtle mental effects may be difficult to detect in them.

Regardless, I needed to find accurate information so that I could address this issue with those who had been exposed and wanted answers. Following mercury history on how policies were made, the economic interests that influenced them, and what data were used in establishing them would prove fascinating and would, I hoped, be helpful to me, my patients, and anyone else concerned about the effects of mercury poisoning on health.

CHAPTER 7

The Summit

TOWARD THE END OF MY YEAR-LONG MERCURY SURVEY of the patients in my private practice of internal medicine, other doctors began sending referrals to me for a mercury consultation. My medical colleagues were seeing similar nonspecific symptoms, with corresponding elevated mercury levels, in some of their patients and suggested they come to me for advice. This brought further opportunity for me to tell my colleagues what I knew, as I would send back a consultation letter that I hoped could be informative for any other patient they might encounter who had a similar range of symptoms. The simple message was that when it came to making a diagnosis for the patient's symptoms, methylmercury was a diagnosis of exclusion. In other words, the symptoms were nonspecific and could be seen in many other diseases or as a result of other contaminants. After other conditions or diseases have been ruled out, mercury should be considered as the cause. It was probably the easiest obtainable diagnosis, based as it was on a simple blood test, and had the most cost-effective treatment of any disease one might otherwise encounter that had roughly similar symptoms. The treatment was simple: Stop the exposure—which in my population meant no fish for at least six months. The important thing was to diagnose it and stop the exposure before any permanent damage occurred.

For the twelve-month interval of the survey that I began in March 2000, I had seen 720 different individuals in my practice and had obtained mercury tests for 123. Some found me through the Internet and the press. I did see some individuals who thought mercury was the cause of their ailments only to discover that other conditions, such as vitamin B6 toxicity, vitamin A toxicity, cancer, endocrine disorders, or hepatitis C, were the more likely source of their discomfort. Not only did I have to become an expert in mercury, but I also had to know all about fish, other heavy metals, omega-3 fatty acids, and the effects of exposure to other contaminants such as polychlorinated biphenyls (PCBs). This also led to my learning as much as I could about toxicants and environmental medicine more generally. I began attending lectures and conferences and reading more about substances that adulterate our environment. Without a grant, I had to be my own secretary, file clerk, researcher, data entry person, and writer. This, of course, was on top of my other roles as mom, wife, cook, doctor, housecleaner, and grocery shopper.

During the period of my survey, one case in particular had always stuck in my mind. A pleasant, well-educated couple, whom I will call the Patels, brought their son to me for consultation after seeing the 20/20 show. Their son, Ajay, who had just turned seven, had been declining in his social skills, memory, fine motor skills, and school performance since the age of three, they said. He also complained of stomachaches, headaches, and lethargy off and on during that time; and his mother mentioned that he would turn red in warm bathwater. He had been thoroughly examined and tested multiple times by neurologists and had completed extensive neuropsychiatric testings. The working diagnosis was Asperger's syndrome, which is essentially a minor form of autism, but the diagnosis was still not certain.

Ajay had been eating albacore and ahi steaks and canned albacore since the age of two, although his parents did not eat much fish themselves. His mother explained, "He loves tuna. We were told it was good for you, so we gave him all he wanted. We have a freezer full of tuna." As his parents and I spoke in my consultation room, the boy did not speak much and demonstrated a mild lack of coordination, bumping his head accidentally several times on my desk while he wandered and crawled about in the room. Compared to other seven-year-olds, he seemed distant, content in his own world, and seldom made eye contact.

His mother said that she was from northern India, where she did not eat fish growing up, but her husband was from southern India and ate a lot of salmon and other smaller fish and shellfish, though not much tuna. The Patel family had their hair tested for mercury. The parents' measures were near the EPA's acceptable level, but Ajay had a hair mercury level of about 15 mcg/g—about fifteen times higher than the EPA guidelines. The EPA says a "safety factor" of 10 was built into its guidelines to keep children well within a statistically calculated margin of safety. But for this child, that safety factor seemed to be easily surpassed.

I have continued to follow this youngster's progress. In 2001 he stopped his mercury intake, and, subsequently, he not only stopped his mental decline but improved in many ways. He no longer had chronic headaches and stomachaches; he could name all the children in his class; and he was more social, active, and aware. But he will most likely need special education and help for the rest of his life, as he still has difficulty with schoolwork, language skills, and social skills. We may never be able to "prove" that mercury or other contaminants harmed him, but we can say that his profile was "consistent" with the mercury effects seen in some children with comparable exposure levels.

After the 20/20 program, the doctors' dining room continued to be a source of lively conversation, as my colleagues would ask for updates. "You should save people's hair to prove your results," one elderly physician colleague insisted one day. I replied that it was not a criminal investigation—at least not that I was aware of. I had been using a good lab, and I rechecked the levels when significant results occurred. At that moment, Dr. Wiviott came in with a big pile of tofu and turkey on his salad and sat down. All eyes focused on his plate. Dr. Wiviott just looked over at me, shrugged his shoulders, and said, "Well, it can't hurt to exercise precaution in one's diet." The room erupted with laughs and exclamations of, "Yeah, Hightower, you ruined my diet."

Not only did my colleagues continue to sit with me, but I was also approached by the San Francisco Medical Society (SFMS), of which I was a member, to write a paper on mercury directed at the general practitioner for the *San Francisco Medicine* magazine. I was being given an opportunity to speak in a public medical forum, I realized, and I did not take the responsibility lightly.

San Francisco Medicine published my first article on mercury, "The

Danger of Mercury Poisoning from Fish," in its March 2001 issue.[1] It was received well by my colleagues, and it gave me an opportunity to extend the discussion of mercury toxicity among more of my peers.

The following month, in April 2001, I finally got to meet Kathryn (Katy) Mahaffey of the U.S. EPA office. She came out to investigate what I had found among my patients. Katy got her start in the EPA when the issue of lead toxicity was being fought. Through her experiences, she had become well equipped to take on the mercury issue and play a leading role in the EPA's 1997 *Mercury Study Report to Congress*.[2] She was a fifty-something woman with brown, shoulder-length hair and an air of "I am on important serious business," yet she was approachable, pleasant, and cautious.

Mahaffey's interest in my study seemed evident immediately—not by any emotional display, but by her questions about my avid fish-eating patients. She asked about their occupations, their age, gender, and ethnicity. She told me what she believed was important about my data and explained how individuals in charge of overseeing fish at the FDA were pressured and could be influenced by the fishing industry. She confirmed my suspicion that the FDA thought my population did not exist. "What will the FDA think when my data show otherwise?" I asked her. "They will be astonished," she replied. "This is powerful data."

I explained why I felt so strongly that my patients were affected by the mercury and told her of my intention to keep my new paper simple and let the data stand on their own. I should "just stick to the numbers," she agreed. "We know people have symptoms, but this [cause and effect] was harder to prove," she said. "I need your numbers, Jane. I cannot push the FDA any harder until I have your numbers."

The FDA still had to be convinced that there were people in the United States who were at risk—that was clear. I thought of Dr. Seuss's *Horton Hears a Who*, wherein the tiny people in Horton's dust speck scream, "We are here!" But only Horton hears their cries. It was a bit like that for me with my mercury patients, who also needed to be heard. Someone at the EPA was willing to listen. Why wasn't the FDA?

Mahaffey and I discussed the CDC's recent National Health and Nutrition Examination Survey, which showed that about 10 percent of the population had blood levels of mercury greater than 5.0 mcg/l, the EPA guideline—but those levels were typically only in the range of 6 to 7 mcg/l and not at the levels I was seeing. This was because high-risk people were not tested in the government report she was talking about. In contrast, of the 116 subjects for whom I had blood level results, 103 (89%) were ≥5.0 mcg/l, 63 (54%) were ≥10 mcg/l, 19 (16%) were ≥20 mcg/l, and 4 were >50 mcg/l. The highest blood level was 89 mcg/l, and the mean was 14.0 mcg/l.[3]

The next morning Mahaffey came with me to the lecture I was giving at morning pediatric grand rounds. Since she did not want to bring attention to herself, she said it would be better not to make a formal announcement prior to her arrival. As it turned out, the doctors did not know who she was, what she was doing there, or what her importance was even after an appropriate introduction was made. I looked at the crowd of about fifty people and saw blank stares. It was highly uncommon for a government official to come to such a lecture, let alone someone from Washington.

After my talk, Katy spoke briefly on how the EPA was gathering data on noncommercial fish and why education of the health care provider and the consumer was important. One of the well-respected elder pediatricians commented, "I am worried about making people hysterical, or sounding like an alarmist." Mahaffey simply said, "Well, we don't have hysteria, nor do we want it, but we certainly have a lot of inertia." He agreed.

After lunch, I took Katy on a tour of some of the San Francisco fish markets and neighborhoods where some of my patients lived and did their shopping. One of the first places we stopped was a popular fish market that catered to San Francisco's finest. Katy pulled out of her bag an enormous 1980s Nikon camera, complete with wide-angle lens, and began taking pictures. She wanted to document the type of fish being sold in our area and how it was being presented to the public.

Many of the regular visitors to this market want privacy and are well enough known that they don't want to be recognized and filmed in a store. They can become quite indignant about pictures. My eyes got big when I saw what Katy was doing, and I looked at the disgruntled man behind the counter, who was about to say something. "She's with me," I quickly said. "She's visiting from out of town. They don't have fish like this where she lives." The man behind the counter eased back and answered some of her questions. He even said of the swordfish, "This one was a good three hundred pounds!" Katy looked astonished and declined his offer to sell her a good-sized steak from it.

We ventured into a Whole Foods supermarket. Katy began quietly taking pictures, and within moments an employee came up and asked her to stop, for reasons that were unclear. We then walked around until we found the fish counter. It was filled with mostly large, predatory fish, but before Katy could take any more pictures, the manager came up to us and kindly but tersely asked us to leave. Grudgingly, we did. But a word of advice for anyone going to fish counters with Katy Mahaffey: Do not take her to the places where you yourself shop.

I was encouraged by Katy's visit to hear that I was doing something that could be helpful in sorting out issues surrounding mercury toxicity. I was also encouraged that there was a high-ranking government employee who truly was watching out for the health of the people.

I was able to publish my survey results, in collaboration with the biostatistician Dan Moore, in *Environmental Health Perspectives*, a journal published by the National Institutes of Health, by November 2002 (print version 2003).[4] The title, "Mercury Levels in High-End Consumers of Fish," was used to take advantage of the double meaning of "high-end." Consumers were not only consuming a "high" amount of fish, the fish they were choosing also cost a "high" amount of money—predators cost more money to catch, and among canned tuna lovers, it was the more expensive chunk white or albacore that seemed to be the mercury problem child, not the chunk light.

The depth of my mercury paper was increased by Gabor Hiller of Specialty Labs. He provided not only good quality control for the mercury tests of the study subjects, but also data that set the study subjects in a larger context. He conducted mercury tests on the blood of randomly selected specimens that his lab was testing for other doctors. He did not know what my results were, and I did not know his until the end. In my own study I selected just for people who ate mercury-laden fish; therefore, the percentage of people over 5 mcg/l was high, 89 percent. His tests were done randomly, and diet was unknown. The percentage 5 mcg/l he obtained was 6 percent, which was consistent with mercury blood levels in general U.S. population studies.

This turned out to be incredibly helpful in assessing the laboratory's ability to properly test for mercury. Since I had such a high percentage of people whose levels were elevated, one might have concluded that there was a problem with the lab. Our quality assurance check indicated that my patients' mercury elevations were indeed real.

Obstetricians Heidi Wittenberg and Leslie Kardos also provided me with information on the mercury levels of twenty-two of their pregnant patients. Because the numbers just kept coming in elevated, we realized quickly that more aggressive prevention was in order for our at-risk population before they became pregnant. There was no clear treatment option. Surely, they could change their diets and get their omega-3 fatty acids from the fish known to be low in mercury, but what do you tell the mother about the health of her baby when she had exposed it unknowingly to a substance known to cause brain damage in the fetus? Pregnant women in our community go out of their way to lead the healthiest lifestyles they can when they are expecting. This includes eating food that is organic and not raw or unpasteurized, not drinking alcohol, not taking illicit drugs or harmful medications, and not being exposed to toxicants if they can be avoided. While scientists were still investigating how much mercury it took to harm the fetus, a larger problem here was that these expectant mothers and others like them were unlikely to be aware of how much mercury was in the fish they were consuming, or of its potential harms. With the obstetricians sharing their pregnant patients' mercury levels with me, it became clear that public education on the mercury issue was needed and the elevated numbers added urgency to my work.

The presentations I'd given, the mercury paper's publication, and the interest of Katy Mahaffey at EPA were beginning to lead to more requests to discuss the mercury issue. Katy invited me to present my data at a meeting of mercury experts, to take place in Vermont in October 2002. A native Californian, I jokingly asked, "Vermont? Do I have to get a passport?" She laughed and said, "No, that's Maine."

So off I went to New England for the first time, and after a full day's travel I was already missing my boys and my husband. I had never been away from them for that long, let alone overnight. I settled in to my room and looked over my notes for the talk the next day. I knew I needed to nail it. To date, my world had been that of other doctors, my patients, and occasionally someone from the news media, aside from Katy Mahaffey. This was my first face-to-face introduction to people who had specialized in some of the issues surrounding mercury toxicity.

When I arrived at the conference the next morning, there were fifty people or so eagerly getting coffee and talking to one another. If I had been asked a year prior, I would have said there probably weren't more than ten people who were interested in this subject. Many of the people here represented large organizations of some type, whether government, public health, or nongovernment. They were friendly and seemed to be familiar with one another and each other's organizations. It was obvious I was a newcomer.

As I tried to take a seat in the back of the room, I was plucked from the crowd and escorted to my chair. The woman in charge of the arrangements smiled and said, "You can't hide now. Your seat is with the rest of the panel up at the front." She pointed to where she had placed a large white placard with my name on it.

The other speakers were given twenty to thirty minutes to present, but I was granted forty minutes. There were talks from a public health perspective on mercury issues in humans, mercury levels in fish, nutritional survey results, and the like. Then it was my turn. Most of the speakers were PhD scientists from the Midwest or the East Coast and very knowledgeable about their subject. I would be the only one giving information on clinical data obtained in the private setting of a doctor's office.

Public health surveys, while having important uses, were often emotionally superficial or downright sterile. Having to hide the identity of the study participants, you could lose track sometimes and forget you were talking about people. Such surveys were typically very general and lacked the nuance and telling personal detail who can only come from in-depth interviews. The data points in my work might be identified only by a number, but I knew the people corresponding to those numbers.

By the end of my talk, I was bombarded with many good questions, and I clearly could tell that these scientists were enthusiastic and hungry for more information. Many of them were studying populations in other countries, such as Canadian Indian tribes, the Faroese, and people in South America. Some were public health officials who were in the process of surveying their own communities. We all quickly realized that the very poor and the wealthy are often missed in risk-assessment equations, as they are usually not amenable to government surveys, and in this instance, it might be precisely those groups who were most at risk.

When I returned to the conference the next morning, people were standing around their chairs, coffee in hand, talking or reading the newspaper. They began turning toward me, offering congratulations, shaking my hand, and telling me, "Good job." I thought I had certainly beamed to another universe when someone said, "Did you see Headline News on TV? The ticker tape at the bottom announced your study, and you are in the paper today."

I was speechless. I had made it through some sort of wormhole, for sure. I had previously felt so isolated in my own world. Before the meeting, I hadn't realized there was an army of experts in mercury that were outside my sphere. I concluded that there were two parallel universes here. One was that of a physician's experience (me, in this case) and patients who were directly affected by mercury toxicity, the other was that of formal institutions—government and nongovernment organizations and industry. First contact had been made, and now we had a summit meeting. How to inform the people would be a greater challenge. How do you explain to people that their fish contains a feared poison, but it is okay to eat it in small amounts . . . maybe—we are still unsure.

I was certainly excited to meet the many people at the conference and looked forward to learning more from their papers and expertise. They knew that there were people in the general population who would be at risk through their diet if they chose the higher-mercury fish and consumed them regularly. They did not know how prevalent the problem would be, though, as the high-end consumer had not been included in any appreciable numbers in reports of the CDC or the FDA. Katy Mahaffey at EPA had no inhibitions about reporting on such a population, though, and was genuinely concerned about my population being at risk. The FDA seemed to be missing in action. What forces, I wondered, lay behind its reluctance to address adequately the effects of mercury on health?

CHAPTER 8

Feeling the Heat in Mercury Politics

FROM THE BEGINNING OF MY EXPERIENCE, how the FDA came up with its mercury and fish consumption advisories had been a mystery. The 1997 *Mercury Study Report*, on which Kathryn (Katy) Mahaffey was principal author, blamed most of the ongoing mercury pollution on coal-fired power plants, and Mahaffey was the one who recognized there would be people at risk from consuming the larger fish predators with higher mercury levels. Her report also pointed out a critical link: that power company pollution contributed to fish contamination. Two strong industries would now have to contribute to solutions—or say no solutions were needed.[1]

On December 20, 2000, the EPA determined that it was "appropriate and necessary" to regulate coal- and oil-fired power plants under the Clean Air Act, because they were the largest domestic source of mercury emissions, which presented significant hazards to public health and the environment. The FDA and EPA went on to announce a fish advisory on January 12, 2001, the day *20/20* aired the mercury story.[2] This union between the two agencies was not complete, though, as the FDA still did not render an opinion as to what blood mercury level was safely tolerated by humans, and the EPA thought the advisory should be expanded to include other medium- to high-mercury fish. The advisory called for women of childbearing age, pregnant women, nursing mothers, and small children not to eat swordfish, tilefish, king mackerel, or shark.

In 2000, the FDA had posted an advisory on its Web site, dated 1995, entitled "Mercury in Fish: Cause for Concern?" The first sentence read like an advertisement for two species: "Swordfish and shark taste great—especially grilled or broiled." The FDA did list symptoms that are seen with methylmercury poisoning, such as numbness and tingling sensations around the lips, fingers, and toes (paresthesia), stumbling gait, difficulty with articulating words, tunnel vision, impaired hearing, generalized muscle weakness, fatigue, headache, irritability, and inability to concentrate; but there was no direct discussion of a level of exposure that might begin to bring on these symptoms. Advice at that time finally came on page four: Pregnant women and women of childbearing age who may become pregnant, should limit their consumption of shark and swordfish to no more than once a month (no serving size was given). Other people should limit their consumption of fish species that had methylmercury levels of around 1 mcg/g (parts per million, or ppm) to about seven ounces per week. The FDA went on to say that consumption advice was unnecessary for the top ten seafood species—canned tuna, shrimp, pollock, salmon, cod, catfish, clams, flatfish, crabs, scallops.[3] My patients, though, had had elevated mercury levels from consuming the "no advisory necessary fish" and others and they had many of the symptoms listed by the FDA that can be seen with mercury toxicity.

Because the mercury advisory could only be found buried on a Web site, the FDA seemed to be providing it as a mere formality and not really for the purpose of helping the consumer. According to the California Public Health Department, Katy Mahaffey of EPA, and the FDA itself, the FDA based its advisories on two assumptions: first, that the U.S. population did not consume enough fish for mercury to be of concern; and second, that the mercury content in commercial fish was not high enough to be hazardous. At the same time, the FDA said to limit shark and swordfish consumption because of their mercury content. Mahaffey disagreed with the FDA stand, and she continued to draw criticism from the fishing industry, the FDA, and other government agencies for her view that there were people in the nation who ate a lot of fish and needed to have reliable and readily available advice to avoid overexposure. The coal-fired power companies in the United States resisted as well, and continued to deny that their mercury emissions had much to do with mercury in fish.

Despite the FDA's opinion in 2000, I continued to find evidence of high fish consumption. What events led to the FDA's mercury regulations, who did the testing, and on whom or what were still questions for which I could not find answers. Why were physicians and consumers so ill informed about mercury consumption? Why did the EPA say that less than 5 mcg/l of mercury in blood was our protective level, while the authorities in the California Public Health Department told me that you could have a level of up to 200 mcg/l with no ill effects? As for the FDA, neither at that time nor even at the time of this writing in 2008, have I found a standard for human blood levels on its Web site. That was particularly disturbing because, as mentioned previously, the FDA had jurisdiction over all of commercial fishing; the EPA, with its more stringent stands, oversaw only noncommercial fishing.

Never had I seen such a discrepancy over a health issue, so I decided to look further into this subject myself. I felt I should summon my colleagues into action, as well, if ill effects were showing up with doses far lower than what the FDA and the California Public Health Department had deduced. I hoped my colleagues would then inform their patients of relevant information. Furthermore, physicians themselves were an at-risk group, though few realized it. Curiously, it would turn out to be my Jewish physician colleagues who, as a group, held the records in my practice for the highest mercury levels. Many among them, I discovered, ate canned albacore tuna almost every day from their hospital's cafeteria, and then for dinner often ate other fish that were high on the food chain. This was especially true for those who were trying to eat a kosher diet. (Any lox one consumes probably has little effect; the mercury in salmon is minimal compared to that in large fish like tuna and swordfish.)

Bodybuilders and dieters who consumed large quantities of canned albacore tuna and other large fish were also on the top of the mercury gauge among patients in my practice. One young medical student had been on a bodybuilding program and consumed two to four cans of albacore tuna per day. He began having symptoms such as stomach upset, trouble concentrating, memory loss, fatigue, muscle aches, insomnia, and feelings of depression. His hair level was 44 mcg/g—forty-four times higher than it should have been. He stopped eating canned albacore, and many of his symptoms improved, but it is too early to tell whether he will obtain complete resolution of the neurological symptoms. Others I found to be particularly at risk were those who relied heavily on fish for their main protein source. Some ethnic groups, such as Asians, Pacific Islanders, and some Native Americans, also were known to consume a relatively large quantity of fish. Then there were the folks who just loved fish. I refer to all these groups collectively as fishatarians.

If physicians who were at risk could not recognize the problem in themselves, they would be unlikely to recognize it in their patients, I realized. Having the American Medical Association, California Medical Association (CMA), and the San Francisco Medical Society (SFMS) actively interested was therefore critical for bringing about physician recognition of possible mercury symptoms in themselves and their patients. Thanks to my colleague Josh Rassen, MD, who suggested the idea, I decided to write a resolution for our medical society to recognize methylmercury as a health hazard in food.

With the help of Steve Heilig of SFMS, we were able to convert a second letter I'd written to Senator Dianne Feinstein from November 2002 into a resolution.[4] The first "whereas" identified methylmercury as a well-documented toxic substance for which there had been no controlled trials using human subjects to address its safety. The second "whereas" referenced my published paper in *Environmental Health Perspectives*, which identified high-end consumers of fish and subsequent elevated mercury levels. I also mentioned that those fish consumers had been suffering from symptoms indicative of mercury exposure and that many had incurred significant health bills in search of the source of their symptoms. The third clause indicated that my population of patients obtained their mercury only from fish that were under FDA jurisdiction. The last "whereas" indicated that in my study, women of reproductive age and pregnant women were found to have levels considered unsafe for a developing fetus; some patients, including children, were within the current FDA guidelines for fish consumption but in excess of the guidelines established by the EPA and the National Academy of Sciences. In addition, the majority of the study patients had mercury levels that could increase their risk of myocardial infarction and cardiovascular death, according to recent studies published in *Circulation*, an American Heart Association journal, and a recent report in the *New England Journal of Medicine*.[5]

The four "resolves" of the resolution were simple. In the first I asked for the testing of mercury in fish to be continued by the appropriate agencies and for laboratory reporting of the results to be updated and kept consistent with EPA and National Academy of Sciences standards. The second was that results and advisories of any mercury testing of fish be made readily available where fish were sold and on labels of packaged or canned fish. Third, food sources that contained significant levels of methylmercury should be excluded from federally funded programs such as the Women Infants Children (WIC) program and free school lunch programs. Finally, the matter of mercury contamination should be referred for national action.

The SFMS unanimously passed the full resolution in 2003.[6] The CMA posed a different problem, however. After I presented my resolution to the committee at the annual conference in March 2003, I stood for questions. The first comment was, "Even the people selling the fish don't know what the fish are, let alone anything about mercury. How do we label it?" I replied that it was a problem that needed to be resolved, as some species can have ten to one hundred times more mercury than others. A delegate from Southern California stood up and said, "I have a problem with the part about canned tuna, as so many people eat it and this would have an impact on the industry. I and my committee read the author's paper and feel more information would be needed to make a decision."

As a physician, he should be protecting public health and not be concerned about the tuna industry, I thought to myself. And then I realized he might actually be an integral part of that industry. I countered by mentioning the evidence I'd brought forward: I provided the committee with the Florida Department of Agriculture numbers for mercury content in canned tuna as well as numbers from the FDA and the U.S. Tuna Foundation, the lobbying group for the tuna industry. I also pointed out that methylmercury in a can was no less toxic than methylmercury that was fresh from the catch of the day. The issue of mercury-laden seafood should not be ignored just because the tuna was in a can and had big business supporting it.

When I got back to my chair, an elderly doc leaned over and said, "That was an exquisite presentation, whoever you are."

After the session, I followed my associate, Dr. William (Bill) Andereck, our San Francisco CMA representative to where the CMA delegates would hear the resolutions. It was an enormous room, with name tags on tables set up in long rows and huge movie screens high on the walls. He assured me that as one of the delegates, he would follow the resolution through, but his parting words were, "Remember, resolutions are written by people who care too much for people who do not care at all."

While the CMA was meeting, another issue of mercury and fish was making news in the state. This was California's Proposition 65. According to this statute, any time a substance was known to the State of California to cause cancer, birth defects, or reproductive harm, a warning had to be given if there were a danger of exposure, so people could decide themselves about the risk they wanted to assume.

Shortly after my paper was published, some nongovernmental organizations that had been following the mercury in fish issue for more than three years, including the Natural Resources Defense Council (NRDC), the Turtle Restoration Project, the Mercury Policy Project, and California Communities Against Toxics, had begun pushing for Proposition 65 warnings about mercury to be instituted for restaurants and grocery stores. In the initial documents filed, my paper was used as the proof of our community's exposure. California attorney general Bill Lockyer had also cited the paper as evidence of the people's exposure in a press release on mercury and Proposition 65.[7]

I had accepted an NRDC invitation to give a short presentation on my findings to the California deputy attorney general and some others at a Proposition 65 meeting in March, coincidentally on the same date my resolution was under discussion by the CMA. Five minutes before the meeting, I managed to reach Bill Andereck. I tersely asked, "Bill, I am about to go into the elevator for my meeting, what got passed?"

"Essentially, three of four resolves passed as written," he said. The WIC resolve was not passed because they just were not ready for it. He then explained, "Some guy got up and asked that the word 'pelagic' be added to the resolution. No one knew what pelagic was, so that didn't happen. I got to speak last, and I finally said to the delegation that . . . all this press about methylmercury was scaring people. We need warning labels to identify the good fish to eat, and that was it; they passed all the rest."[8]

The first person to speak at my meeting was Jane Williams of California Communities Against Toxics, who told of a previous mercury suit against the tuna industry that had ended in a 1998 agreement that the tuna companies would keep mercury levels in canned tuna less than 0.25 mcg/g. Her organization recently tested fifty samples of canned tuna for mercury concentrations and discovered that the industry was in violation of that agreement. She said, "I know that the tuna king will fight to the death to keep labels off his cans of tuna, but our testing shows the need for them."

When it was my turn to speak, I began with "What I have to bring to the table today is my knowledge, my paper, my patients, and the California Medical Association." After the initial shock in the room, Deputy Attorney General Sue Fiering was especially pleased and quite interested, as, evidently, this was the first time physicians had taken any significant stand on this health issue in California.

Jane Williams explained to the group that the Tuna Foundation hired a lot of consultants. Even the Tuna Foundation's FDA consultants told the Foundation in 1998 that the amount of mercury in canned tuna was rising and that in five to ten years it would be more of a problem. The tuna industry was adamant that no labeling should take place. Jane said she had come to this meeting to ask the attorney general to help in enforcing the previous settlement, in which the tuna industry was to keep the mercury levels less than 0.25 mcg/g.

The meeting gave me a bit of insight as to what was going on behind the scenes. Still, Jane Williams and Sue Fiering met privately for a longer period. Only later did I learn the details of a confidential agreement between the Tuna Foundation and Williams's organization.

Evidently, two meetings had taken place in March and May of 1998 among the tuna industry, the California attorney general, and several others, which had decided the fate of California consumers in regard to their exposure to mercury in the ensuing years.

As for my CMA resolution that had passed, it was slated soon to be presented to the American Medical Association. But the Southern California delegation was still fighting to keep mercury labels off canned tuna and to keep canned tuna in the WIC and free school lunch programs. It wasn't difficult to figure out where the prime sympathies of this delegation lay. The canned tuna industry had an exclusive deal with these federally funded programs and was not about to lose it. If a neurotoxin was identified on canned tuna labels, pregnant women and others might be deterred from consuming it. Worse yet, they might just demand a healthier alternative from their government program.

The important thing was that the CMA now recognized methylmercury as a hazard in fish and was the first delegation to do so. Physicians would no longer have to feel alone or out on a limb when considering mercury in the differential diagnosis of their patients. Because of fear of being labeled as a less-than-superb clinician, or of litigation, physicians were often slow to adopt new policy unless their peers overwhelmingly accepted it. The mercury issue was different, though. There was a lot of information in the literature, enough to warrant advisories by federal government agencies. But the information was not getting to the consumer or the health care community. Something just wasn't right.

The CMA was certainly applauded by most people and criticized by industry for passing my mercury resolution. Since it was decided that the resolution would go to the AMA for further action, the issue had a chance for national acceptance. But with the AMA, the industry had more time to interfere in the process. Because I was not an official California delegate, I would still not be allowed on the floor of the AMA convention when the discussions took place, nor would industry. The bartering would certainly be a behind-the-scenes effort. I therefore called a few physicians in other states to support the CMA resolution.

By May of 2003, I was receiving many phone calls, e-mails, and letters from mercury-concerned individuals, the media, nongovernment organizations, physicians, and patients. Jane Allen of the *Los Angeles Times* was one of the first in a series who asked me to comment on the latest article released that year from the Seychelles study, which apparently showed no adverse effects to infants exposed in-utero to methylmercury through their mother's consumption of fish.

In my endeavor to gain knowledge about and understanding of the mercury issue, I had learned early on that there were two studies in progress on methylmercury exposure through fish consumption, each conducted to assess the lowest discernible effects on children. One study was ongoing in the Republic of Seychelles, conducted by researchers at the University of Rochester, New York, and the Seychelles government. The other was ongoing in the Faroes Islands, conducted by researchers at the University of Southern Denmark and Harvard. The Seychelles researchers continued to conclude that there were no effects seen in the children they studied, while the Faroes study did show effects. Industry groups, such as those in support of coal-burning power plants and commercial fishing, used the Seychelles study as evidence that eating mercury was not harmful and mercury emissions from coal were not a problem. The Faroes was the study most quoted by nongovernment organizations in support of advisories to protect the consumer from overexposure.

In June 2003, my resolution recognizing mercury as a health hazard in food was to be presented by Judy Mates, MD, our CMA delegate to the national AMA meeting. On the day our resolution was to be heard, she sent an e-mail from Chicago in a near panic, asking, "What is this about a 'new directive that mercury causes no harm'?" I had not heard of such a "directive," and I knew then that we were being blocked or opposed by someone. There was no new directive. There was a new paper by the Seychelles researchers, but it addressed only limited aspects of mercury toxicity. Dr. Mates had worked for years in various capacities in the AMA, CMA, and SFMS, and she said she had never had anything like this happen before. When there had been opposition to a resolution, those opposed identified themselves. This time, however, she could get no further information on who was introducing the notion of a "new directive." She reiterated, "Someone has told the AMA, possibly by e-mail or letter, that there was this new directive, but no one seems to want to tell me more than that."

I called some of my mercury colleagues to discuss the directive given to the AMA. One of them in turn faxed to me a presentation that Philip Davidson, a Seychelles researcher, was to give soon entitled "From Loaves to Fishes."[9] The sender of the fax thought I would want to know that in the acknowledgments of this upcoming presentation by Davidson, it stated that a grant was paid to him by EPRI. What was EPRI?

EPRI was the Electric Power Research Institute—one of the biggest lobbying entities for the power companies, including those that held coal-burning power plants. Coal-fired power plants were implicated as a major producer of mercury pollution in the air, of course, and were thought to be a significant contributor to the mercury problem in fish. There was an ongoing debate as to just how much of an impact these plants had on the environment. But mercury-polluting industries would have an interest in knowing the extent to which their emissions were thought to cause an increase in mercury in the environment, fish, and humans, with possibly harmful effects, and would not be happy about a bad outcome in any study conducted. Philip Davidson was one of the main researchers involved with the Seychelles study and was affiliated with the University of Rochester, the university where most of the Seychelles researchers were located. In my Internet searches, I had crossed the path of the University of Rochester and mercury before. A 1998 university Web page, for example, cited a paper entitled "Commercial Fish: Eat Up Despite Low Levels of Mercury."[10]

If EPRI was funding any part of a study (or giving money to the researchers) that was trying to discern how much methylmercury from fish was harmful, we would want to know more details. Experts in the field often consult for both sides, and whether the funding entities have influence over what is studied, how, and what conclusions are derived in the end is a problem the scientific community has always faced. Further investigation over the funding for the Seychelles study was therefore warranted.

As a physician, I use the scientific literature to help inform, diagnose, and educate my patients. Competing financial interests can bias papers in science in many ways. These competing interests are supposed to be declared so that others reading the scientific papers can take the possibility of bias into consideration. Physicians are especially sensitive to these conflicts, as drug companies pay for major studies that give us direction on medications used in the treatment of our patients.

The next day, Judy Mates called again and told me of her effort to have the resolution heard on the floor of the AMA convention. "Someone has convinced the committee that there was this new directive, that mercury was not harmful," she told me. She went on to say that many at the AMA convention did not even know that the EPA and FDA provided warnings about mercury in fish. They just did not have enough knowledge to rule on the resolution. She felt that the council would need more information about the human effects of methylmercury in fish and suggested that I flood them with it.

So much for the FDA's "widely available warnings." Clearly, the physicians in this country were in need of some education on this subject. If the AMA, and ultimately the practicing physicians, did not know about the possibility of their patients being overexposed to methylmercury with possible harm to them as a result, the patients would not be properly diagnosed. I recall a woman who came to see me from Minnesota for a consultation about her blood mercury level of 35 mcg/l and various symptoms. The patient had asked her doctor for the test. What had the doctor told her about the test? "She told me I was weird," the patient replied. I assured her that she was not the only person who came to me with that dubious distinction. I gave her reassurance that she was indeed normal, but that she was being exposed to too much methylmercury. She changed her diet immediately and all but eliminated her exposure. Only time will tell if all her symptoms will resolve completely.

Because someone was spreading a rumor of a new directive to the AMA, the resolution was forced into the Council of Scientific Affairs for further investigation before it could be brought to the floor, essentially killing it for that year's convention. At that point I thought that if I was going to influence my profession's awareness of the dangers posed by methylmercury, I had better get more involved in matters of governance. The following year I was elected to the board of directors for the San Francisco Medical Society. There seemed to be overwhelming complacency in my profession—to the point that I have heard many businesspeople state that physicians are like cats: They don't lead, they don't follow, and they don't get out of the way.

In the meantime, I called many researchers and mercury experts to request that they provide the AMA with information on methylmercury, and they did. Katy Mahaffey of EPA invited the person in charge of looking at the resolution for the Council on Scientific Affairs, Barry Dickinson, to the Tampa Mercury Symposium in April 2004, so he could become as informed as possible on methylmercury issues. The AMA even became one of the sponsors for this symposium, along with the FDA and EPA and others. I was an invited lecturer, as well.

Dickinson and the council presented their report to the AMA in June 2004. In their executive summary, they concluded that women who might become pregnant, are pregnant, or are nursing should follow federal, state, and local advisories on fish consumption. Because these advisories may differ, the most protective advisory should be followed. Physicians should assist in educating patients about the relative mercury content of fish and shellfish products and should make them aware of current advisories on fish consumption. Testing of the mercury content of fish should be continued by appropriate agencies, and results should be publicly accessible and reported in a "consumer-friendly format." They went on to say, "Given the limitations of national fish consumption advisories, the FDA also should consider the advisability of requiring that fish consumption advisories and results related to mercury testing be posted where fish, including canned tuna, are sold."[11]

Because I was perplexed about how a rumor could temporarily but effectively derail the AMA from accepting the resolution for vote, I continued my investigation into EPRI and the Seychelles study. I was able to locate another connection of the Seychelles research project with EPRI, in a report from the Joint Institute for Food Safety and Applied

Nutrition (JIFSAN) published in 1998–1999. JIFSAN was a joint research body of the University of Maryland and the FDA. Through this organization, colleagues from the University of Maryland and the University of Rochester cooperated on an eighteen-month pilot study on human neurobehavioral outcomes at age eleven of children who participated in the Seychelles Child Development Study. According to the report, "JIFSAN played a critical role in bringing together the resources to continue this long-term study on the developmental effects of mercury. Funding for the project was provided by the FDA, the Electric Power Research Institute ($486,000), The National Tuna Foundation ($10,000) and The National Fisheries Institute ($5,000)."[12]

I have no objections to anyone giving money for research, and I hope the authors declared this type of money when testifying before Congress, lecturing on the subject, and in their many papers on the Seychelles research project, as it would be considered a conflict of interest. The three private donating entities had a financial interest in the outcome of the study and would likely want to refute the notions that there is too much mercury in some of the fish the public is consuming and that the mercury bellowing out of coal-fired power plants has contributed to the problem. Simply keeping a project going with money, supplies, and so forth and therefore keeping the scientists employed is one way bias can be introduced if investigators are susceptible to it. (That bias is possible, of course, but doesn't in itself mean that it exists.) Donators usually do not want to continue to fund a project whose results would be damaging to their economic survival.

When I received this information on potential conflicts of interest, I did not feel it was my place to challenge the scientists involved in this matter, but it certainly was in the jurisdiction of the nongovernment organizations. I therefore turned the investigation over to the Natural Resources Defense Council (NRDC) in Washington, DC.

Jennifer Sass and Linda Greer led the investigation for NRDC and corresponded with the *Lancet*, then later with the *New England Journal of Medicine*, where the Seychelles researchers had recently published papers about the Seychelles study and a review paper on mercury. Sass and Greer also submitted a letter to the editor, stating that the authors had not revealed their funding in the papers submitted and that this was a violation of the conflict of interest rules for the journals.[13]

Sass's and Greer's letter to the *Lancet* gained a response from Dr. Constantine Lyketsos, a geriatrician at Johns Hopkins and a Seychelles study author and researcher. He wrote, "I have no conflicts of interest that relate to this research, and receive no funding from the fisheries or from any other industries involved in this area." Dr. Gary Myers of the University of Rochester, "on behalf of the Seychelles study group," wrote an even longer reply. He stated, "The National Institute of Environmental Health Sciences (NIEHS) was the sole source of funding for this study, but had no other role. However, as is common with Universities, our group has received support from other government agencies and private research foundations, some of which receive their support from industry (Electric Power Research Institute and the National Fisheries Institute). Those other funding sources played no role in this study nor did they have any influence upon data collection, interpretation, analysis or writing of the manuscript." He then went on to declare the various government grants they received, and none involved industry.[14]

The problems with Dr. Myers's statement were several. Usually the authors have to reveal their funding sources and conflicts of interest when they submit a paper for publication. The customary time frame for many journals is to report any conflicts within three to five years of the study. On Myers's own Web site, he listed in his supported research section a paper that listed EPRI as a coinvestigator from May 2000 to May 2003.[15] This paper involved the Seychelles Child Development project, which has been ongoing since the 1980s. The *Lancet* paper on the Seychelles came out in May 2003 but did not disclose that EPRI had funded part of the Seychelles Child Development Study or that the researchers were given honoraria that would likely be considered a conflict of interest. In May 1999, the Seychelles researchers submitted a paper to *Environmental Health Perspectives* that was solely supported by EPRI.[16] In July 2003, Davidson was receiving money from EPRI directly for a presentation and subsequent report he gave on methylmercury. In other words, EPRI was involved in the funding of the Seychelles project and gave honoraria to one of its authors. Although the authors declared EPRI funding in some of their papers, they did not declare it as a conflict of interest in their concurrent papers, such as the 2003 paper published in the *Lancet* or their 2003 review paper on mercury submitted to the *New England Journal of Medicine*.[17]

Although Dr. Myers felt it was not important to mention his support from the coal-fired power plant lobbying institute to the *Lancet* or *NEJM* or the funding from the National Fisheries and the Tuna Foundation, he removed the EPRI paper he referenced from his Web page, as it was no longer there within several weeks of the beginning of the investigation.

Even though there was direct evidence of an issue with appropriate declaration of funding, those journals decided there was no conflict of interest in this case. An e-mail forwarded to me from Sass and Greer that was allegedly to them from Ms. Abigail Pound of the *Lancet* stated, "In view of the fact that neither group has any conflicts of interest, as suggested by you, we have decided that to publish the exchange is of no benefit to readers."

John Fialka of the *Wall Street Journal* also had difficulty in getting some of the Rochester mercury researchers to disclose their funding sources. When he asked Thomas Clarkson, a long-time mercury investigator and main Seychelles–University of Rochester researcher about EPRI funding to the Seychelles study, Clarkson replied, "While the institute [EPRI] provided some incidental support, the financing for the study came from the U.S. government."[18]

Was there a difference between "incidental support" and "financing"? I could have used some of that "incidental $486,000 support." For my interest in diagnosing and advising patients, the politics of policy-making and the lax funding disclosures of some mercury researchers were beginning to seem like a kind of find-the-money-if-you-can game that was far from reassuring.

CHAPTER 9

The Canadian Mercury Scare

I N SEARCHING FOR THE SOURCE of government standards of mercury's toxicity, I had quickly realized that discussions in the United States on how much mercury would be allowed in commercial fish and how much was considered safe were based on poisoning incidences that to many of the discussants were vague recollections at best. Where, when, and how these poisonings transpired and were studied seemed important to know. In medicine, when making a diagnosis, it is best to collect your own information, as close to the source as you can. This reduces the rate of errors in your conclusions in many ways.

My search led to Canada, where it appears that much of the modern discussion of mercury pollution in North America began, more than thirty-five years ago. Thanks to Professors Patricia and Frank D'Itri, who investigated mercury pollution in Michigan and Canada in the 1970s; Eugene and Aileen Smith, who extensively documented the Minamata disaster, which helped set the context for the discussions; and Barney and Marion Lamm, who kept track of it all, I was able to put some of the pieces together more efficiently than I might have on my own.[1]

In 1969, the Canadian Federal Department of Fisheries and Forestry embargoed commercial fishing catches from Lake Winnipeg, Cedar Lake, the Saskatchewan River, and the Red River in the province of Manitoba because of high levels of mercury. The government set a temporary 0.5 mcg/g ppm action level and decreed that all fish with higher mercury levels were unsafe for human consumption. Initially, more than one million pounds of fish with mercury levels 5–10 mcg/g were confiscated and destroyed. At that time, a man named Norvald Fimreite predicted that mercury levels in fish would also be high in the waterways of neighboring Ontario and Quebec provinces, where two-thirds of the Canadian chlor-alkali plants were located. His conclusion was based on responses from an array of company officials who estimated that, on average, a half pound of mercury was discharged into the waterways for each ton of chlorine produced, or a total of approximately 200,000 pounds of mercury per year. Fimreite's findings, as relayed by the D'Itris, were substantiated in Ontario province when the Water Resources Commission surveyed mercury losses from pulp and paper mills as well as chlor-alkali plants. The Reed (now Dryden) Paper Company alone, it was later alleged, had dumped 10 tons of mercury into the waterways.[2] Dumping in Canada was, in fact, commonplace, as there were few regulations against it on the books or penalties that would likely be incurred for any harm it caused.

By the fall of 1969, both Fimreite and George Kerr, the Ontario minister of energy and resources, sent samples to be tested of fish from Lake St. Clair, which lies between the state of Michigan on the western side and the province of Ontario on the eastern side. Results showed that mercury in the fish was above the acceptable tolerance level of 0.5 mcg/g. The culprit in this contamination was Dow Chemical Company of Sarnia, Ontario. According to a Canadian Broadcast Company (CBC) investigative report, the Ontario government acknowledged that mercury had been leaking from the plant as far back as 1949.[3]

The Canadian government acted swiftly to protect its people from further exposure, and within a week of the findings, eighteen thousand pounds of walleye were seized from commercial fishermen on the Ontario side of Lake St. Clair. The next day the Canadians banned all commercial and sportfishing on their side of the lake. Dow Chemical later claimed the company immediately began a "crash cleanup program," as well. St. Clair was thought to be one of the best tourism fishing lakes in North America, and the impact on commercial and sportfishing and tourism was devastating. In one CBC interview a fisherman said he already had his fish tagged and loaded on the truck when the order came down. "We were closed up with just a telephone call," he said.[4]

The problem with the 0.5 action level, Frank D'Itri pointed out, was that it was based on average fish consumption and did not take into consideration subpopulations of people who consumed more, such as subsistence fishermen who lived in those polluted areas.[5] The difference in exposure in consuming six ounces (170 grams) of 0.5-mcg/g mercury-laden fish once or twice per week compared to consuming that amount every day is considerable. For a 132-pound (60-kilogram) person, this would be the difference between a blood level of about 18 and one of 64 mcg/l. Even 18 is too high, though, when looking at my patients' levels, their symptoms, and the cardiac literature. The Indian peoples of the area were subsistence fishermen, and telling them not to eat local fish would be like telling them to starve. For those consuming daily fish, it would be important to have the mercury in it be ten times less to prevent their bodies from accumulating it. Most likely, no fish that low in mercury were available in those polluted bodies of water.

The results of the mercury tests also led the Ontario government to issue orders, in February 1970, to eleven companies to stop dumping mercury into the waterways. Fimreite's findings, which included testing fish, birds, and other wildlife on multiple waterways in Canada, were made public several weeks later. Northern pike tested up to 28 mcg/g of mercury, walleye at 20 mcg/g, and bass at 10 mcg/g. These levels were certainly higher than many fish tested in Japan's Minamata mercury crisis, and they were confirmed by the Canadian Government Fisheries Board. The Canadian Food and Drug Directorate then formally advised the U.S. FDA of the mercury problem, the U.S. Embassy in Ottawa informed the secretary of state, as well, and officials on both sides of the lake began studying mercury's impact.[6]

Although it appeared that the Canadian government had everything under control, a different story began to emerge through the media. In November 1974, a Canadian news agency obtained a 1972 document entitled "The Public Health Significance of Methylmercury" that had been prepared for the Ontario cabinet by a branch of the Ontario Department of Public Health. It stated, "In the Wabigoon-English river system, levels in the fish are amongst the highest recorded in North America and are comparable with those found in Japan." This river system stretches across the middle of the two provinces of Saskatchewan and Manitoba and is far from Lake St. Clair and St. Clair River. By August 1974, the report had still not been released. When asked about the mercury levels in St. Clair, George Kerr, Ontario's minister of the environment at the time, responded in a CBC November 1974 interview, "The statement that the levels are higher than the situation in Japan is a damn lie."[7]

Linking the Minamata disaster, whose harms concurrently were being so bitterly contested in court and on the streets of Japan, to conditions in Canada would certainly send a strong message to the Canadian government. But this was not the first time the government had heard that comparison. Dr. Gordon J. Stopps, a provincial health official, stated in 1971 of the Wabigoon-English River system, "There isn't an expert in the world who would say those fish are fit to eat." In his opinion, "eating one 7-ounce fish fillet from the Wabigoon-English River system per day for three weeks would increase the mercury blood levels to the range at which some persons were poisoned at Minamata."[8]

Were the levels as high as they had been in Minamata? I wanted to find out for myself. But obtaining the above referenced 1972 report was a challenge for me, as well, since the Canadian government documents librarian did not seem to have it, and the university that the librarian said once had it no longer did. Thanks to two resort owners turned activists, Barney and Marion Lamm, I was able to obtain a copy through Harvard.[9]

In this Ontario Department of Health report, it was disclosed that blood mercury levels of individuals eating fish out of the St. Clair River, which feeds into Lake St. Clair and the English River, ranged from 10 to 358 mcg/l. The average umbilical cord blood for twenty-nine babies was 21 mcg/l.[10] These levels certainly are high and are in a range where one could see symptoms of overt methylmercury toxicity.

The day after the radio program accused the Canadian government of not disclosing the report when it was completed two years earlier, the revelation was the subject of a heated argument in the Ontario legislature. A few selections will give the flavor of just how some members of the government were taking care of their citizens at the time.[11]

When asked about the report on the English and St. Clair Rivers, Minister of Health F. S. Miller stated, "Mr. Speaker, to the best of my knowledge there may be a federal report that's not public. . . . Now there were no other formal reports. There are working documents within the ministries, I assume, but I know of no working document that even specifically relates to that area. I know of at least one that relates to health problems related to mercury, for example, but not one that deals with the Wabigoon or English river type of system."

Mr. R. F. Nixon: "Is the minister, then, unable to indicate to the House why this programme and the researchers reporting through it, would indicate that information from Ontario was unaccountably impeded?"

Mr. L. C. Henderson (of Lambton): "Bunch of Liberals!"

Mr. R. F. Nixon: "Almost everybody is."

Hon. Mr. Miller: "I have a letter from the Federal people saying just the opposite; that in fact they appreciated the co-operation of my ministry in handing them information."

Mr. Nixon: "Can the Minister then assure the House that the implications in the programme, which indicate there is a serious and continuing threat to the health of the Indian communities, are in error?"

Mr. Miller: "No, Mr. Speaker, I wouldn't go so far, because I am concerned and we have been concerned about the threat to the health of the Indian people from mercury."

Later in this report:

Mr. Miller: "We have set, arbitrarily, 100 parts per billion [mcg/l] as the maximum level of methylmercury we would like to have in the blood of a human being. That's based on assumption: The lowest level that we've ever been able to assume affected the health of a human being was 200 parts per billion of methylmercury. That was found in Japan, by what we call extrapolation, not by actual tests, at a time when testing procedures were not particularly accurate for methylmercury. . . . If we find somebody with 100 parts per billion we refer them to the federal health agencies for treatment or examination."

Mr. Lewis: "May I ask the Minister of Health, does he or does he not have in his possession a report dated Feb. 18, 1972, and entitled, 'The Public Health Significance of Methylmercury,' put out by the environmental health services branch, public health division, Ministry of Health, which contains the observation that mercury levels of fish in the Wabigoon and English River systems are the highest recorded in North America and comparable to Japan? If there is such a report, why is that report not a public document?"

Mr. Miller: "First of all, that is the working document I referred to, and I said there were some working documents in my possession."

Some Honorable Members: "Oh, oh."

Mr. Lewis: "A working document? I see. Everything is suppressed around here under the title of working documents."

Mr. Miller: "It was not suppressed in any sense at all."

Mr. Lewis: "It wasn't? Where is it?'

Mr. Miller: "I have it right here in my hand at this moment.'

Mr. Singer: "Will the Minister table it?"

Interjections by Honorable Members.

Mr. Speaker: "Order, please."

Mr. Miller: "I see no reason why this can't be tabled."

Mr. Lewis: "Put it on the table in this House."

Mr. Singer: "Put it on the table now."

Mr. Miller: "I will, without any question, because I don't see any incriminating evidence in here of the indication—"

Mr. J. E. Stokes (Thunder Bay): "Why not tell the people of Grassy Narrows that?"

Hon. L. Bernier (minister of natural resources): "They have been told."

Mr. Miller: "We have been telling them that—and the Hon. Member knows that."

An Honorable Member: "The Minister is desperate."

Mr. Lewis: "When the minister has a document that contains that kind of information which relates directly to the actual or potential health hazards of all of those who consume fish in the Grassy Narrows and Whitedog reserve areas, how dare he not bring it to public attention for more than two and a half years?"

Interjections from Honorable Members.

Mr. Lewis: "No, seriously, how does he keep it hiding for two and a half years?"

Mr. Miller: "The Hon. Member knows that kind of implication is incorrect."

Mr. Lewis: "The task force report didn't give the working papers."

Mr. Miller: "That was the purpose of that report the member got in April."

Mr. Singer: "Could the minister advise whether any testing has been done, particularly on younger persons, to ascertain tunnel vision, deafness, and other classic symptoms of mercury poisoning; the extent to which those statistics have been gathered; and whether the minister is aware of the fact that the mercury poisoning incident in Japan has caused at least 100 deaths up to this point?"

Mr. Miller: "First of all, Mr. Speaker, that is exactly what we do with the people whose mercury levels are found to be high; they have been tested by the federal people at that point. Our function, and I would say our duty has been to assist in the testing pro-gramme. However, we have been told that it is a federal responsi-bility to look after the health of those people. We have been told that."

Mr. Lewis: "It's nice that health is jurisdictional!"

Mr. Miller: "Look, I don't agree that it should be jurisdictional, and I happen to be telling the federal government that."

An Hon. Member: "Do something!"

Interjections by Honorable Members.

Mr. Speaker: "Order, please."

Mr. Stokes: "Thank you, Mr. Speaker. Is the Minister of Health aware that there was a recommendation from a coroner's jury that a post-mortem should be carried out in any case of death in the Whitedog and Grassy Narrows area where there is any indication of depression? What happened to that recommendation, which his ministry should be concerned about?"

Mr. Miller: "First of all, Mr. Speaker, I am not aware of that coro-ner's recommendation. I will look into it. I can only tell the Hon. Member I am basing these facts not on findings made by doctors whom he might claim were under the control of the Ministry of Health of Ontario, but on findings of doctors who work under the control of the federal government, who have assured us there were no symptoms in the people they have tested."

Mr. Nixon: "I have a question of the Minister of Health on a simi-lar subject. How can the minister tell the House that in his opinion certain federal documents might not have been made public, but the Province of Ontario has made public all information, when in the next breath he refers to a special working document which is not made public? And which contains the incriminating informa-tion that was referred to [in last night's program] in that report?"

Mr. Lewis: "And he didn't intend to make it public."

Mr. Nixon: "How dare he treat the House this way?"

Interjections by Honorable Members.

Mr. Speaker: "Order, please. Does the Hon. Minister have an answer?"

Mr. Miller: "Perhaps not a reply, but I have a pill for the red colour of the member's face which will cut down his blood pressure."

Interjections by Honorable Members.

The above transcript selections tell us this much: There were Indians who had high mercury levels, the water was polluted, individuals in the Canadian government had suppressed the information, and the doctors evaluating the people were using symptom profiles from extrapolated mercury levels based on assumptions found in the Japan poisonings. The Japanese were fighting over what symptoms constituted mercury toxicity as much as the Canadians, in order to sort out all the finger pointing and thus determine the compensation to be awarded to people adversely affected and for the cleanup of the environment. The Indians had high levels of mercury yet were said in the report to be without "symptoms." What types of tests and exams were given to the patients, and who evaluated them, I wondered.

In the early 1970s, as more mercury-polluted waters were discovered, mercury testing in the waterways of North America became widespread. In 1972 the United States and Canada signed the Great Lakes Water Quality Agreement, which "expressed [the] commitment of each country to restore and maintain the chemical, physical, and biological integrity of the Great Lakes Basin Ecosystem, and included a number of objectives and guidelines to achieve those goals."[12]

Unfortunately, while some companies have made great strides in reducing their pollution of the region, many others have not. Lake St. Clair and St. Clair River and the surrounding area have become known as Chemical Valley because of the persistent levels of pollution still found there years later.[13]

When Canada banned commercial fishing on Lakes Erie and St. Clair after it became known that fish there were high in mercury, the sportfishing industry lost millions of dollars in revenue. This led to a "Fish for Fun" program in Canada and in the United States, a "catch and release" program, whereby the fish were returned to the waters after being landed. Signs were posted in Canada that warned of mercury poisoning, but as the sportfishing tourist trade began shutting down, the warning signs also came down. Some reports claimed that lodge owners paid Indians a bottle of whiskey for each sign brought in.[14]

As the resorts and sportfishing lodges were being warned about mercury through telephone calls and written materials, the Ojibway Indians who resided in the areas of Grassy Narrows and Whitedog were allegedly left uninformed. The Reed/Dryden Paper Company had been dumping mercury for years in the waters where the tribe fished. The Ojibway in the region, a community of about a thousand individuals, did not have telephones at that time, nor did they have a written language. They served mainly as fishing guides and domestic help for the fishing lodges and sport fishing industry. Every day, the guides ate the fish out of the polluted waterways. Then, suddenly, there were no more jobs, as the lodges shut down; the unemployment rate jumped from 20 percent to 80 percent. The Indians were told that the fish were laden with mercury and not to eat it as it "may make you sick." When the Indians told their government that they were already sick, chaos began for the Canadians.[15]

With unemployment at 80 percent among the Ojibway, the Canadian government placed the affected people on welfare, but there was no type of government restitution program available for the tribe to further compensate them for the resultant damage to their health and other losses. All industry had to do to avoid restitution was convince the government that the pollution was not harming anyone. Not surprisingly, Reed/Dryden denied that the pollution it dumped into the waterways made the Ojibway ill. A flurry of reports ensued, but the Indians were continually left in the dark, as the Canadian government apparently did not disclose their mercury results to them for a number of years. Other reports in the 1970s attempted to discredit the Indians, claiming that the kids sniffed glue and gas and the adults drank too much, and that therefore it could not be proven that mercury was the cause of their symptoms and illnesses.[16]

As the warning signs were removed, the fishing lodge owners and the government began clearing the air of mercury-scare publicity and opened the lakes and rivers for fishing again, even though the fish were still too contaminated for consumption. By December of 1973, the lodge owners Marion and Barney Lamm had seen enough, however. They were still losing fishing-tourist business because of high methylmercury levels in the fish, and they saw that the Indians affected by mercury were not getting adequate government help. They wrote a letter to Aileen and Eugene Smith asking for help. The Smiths, well versed in the game of pollute, deny, stall, bury, and forget, from their Minamata experience, asked Masazumi Harada, MD, a leading mercury expert in Japan, to come to their aid. Tadeo Takeuchi, known for identifying methylmercury toxicity in cats, offered to help, as well. Both Japanese experts offered to conduct autopsies on Indians who had died but were denied permission to do that by the Canadian government. The challenge of "Show me someone who has died of mercury poisoning" therefore went unanswered. They were able to perform autopsies on some cats that had been eating fish from Northwest Ontario's Wabigoon-English River system downstream from the Dryden paper and pulp mill. It had been noted that the Ojibway's cats were acting strangely and erratically, just as the Minamata cats had done. Takeuchi concluded in the report he submitted in 1976 that the cat findings, along with the symptoms found in the Indians examined, indicated that mercury pollution posed a grave health hazard that should not be ignored.[17] Barney and Marion Lamm were instrumental in helping the Indian people obtain outside help and negotiate with the Canadian government. The D'Itris refer to them as the sacrificial Lamms, as the couple shut down their own fishing lodge as a result of the mercury in the fish and went to great lengths to find answers for their community.[18]

Another man who came to Canada was Thomas Clarkson, a toxicologist from the University of Rochester, who had been developing a polythiol resin under the auspices of Dow Chemical for the purpose of removing mercury from the body—chelating it—at a faster rate than normal. It was said by the CBC that Clarkson came in August 1975 and set up labs for testing in the Whitedog and Grassy Narrows area, but reports I obtained from the Lamm files at Harvard and in Canada contained evidence of Clarkson's prior involvement with Dow, methylmercury pollution and its effects on humans in Canada. Interestingly, the Ontario province filed suit against Dow for its mercury pollution in March 1971.[19]

In February 1971, the Royal Society of Canada held a special symposium entitled "Mercury in Man's Environment," at which Clarkson told how his new resin, 17-B, could remove mercury from the body. He stated that the brain mercury levels in resin-treated animals were five times lower than in untreated animals, and that it was desirable to have the technique available to rapidly remove mercury from the body while the source that contributed to this burden was identified and eliminated.[20]

Clarkson would go on to try to discern whether the Ojibway had signs and symptoms of mercury toxicity at the same time he was collaborating with Dow on his resin. These overlapping roles were similar for Clarkson to those of the Chisso Corporation doctors in Japan. The Minamata case is a good illustration of the problems such dual roles can lead to. One Chisso doctor the Smiths discussed was sympathetic to the people but was not able to help them as well as he might because the company controlled what he was allowed to say and reveal to the public. Other company doctors just remained silent or denied that their company's pollution was causing harm. As the D'Itris recounted, "It was not until July 1969 that an ailing Dr. Hajimé Hosokawa finally testified in court that the famous Cat 400 had confirmed the cause of Minamata Disease at the Chisso factory more than a decade earlier. Out of loyalty to the company he worked for, the conscience-stricken Hosokawa had kept the results secret as the list of victims lengthened over the years."[21]

Just as in Japan, the cat studies in Canada didn't become public quickly. In one CBC report, I found out that the Canadian government allegedly had fed cats fish out of the Wabigoon-English River areas beginning in 1970 to see if the cats would be affected by the mercury content. The results became public only when the Japanese researchers came and were broadcast on CBC television. This 1975 broadcast showed cats struggling to climb and walk under the neurological damage that mercury caused.[22]

The Japanese research team released its report on the Ojibway in 1975, stressing that there "was no doubt of the importance of preventive measures. We must correct our mistake that we limited Minamata Disease to typical, severe cases for political reasons, and prevent the damage before it goes to the irrecoverable stage."[23] Dr. Harada, after examining the Ojibway in the region, found them to have disturbances of eye movement, impaired hearing, sensory disturbance, tunnel vision, tremor, reduced reflexes, difficulty with walking, and trouble speaking. The most common subjective symptom was pain in the limbs. He therefore concluded that although their symptoms could be from other causes, they were consistent with Minamata disease. He was immediately challenged by the Canadian government and the industries affected by evidence of mercury pollution.

Leo Bernier, Ontario's minister of natural resources, responding to the findings of the Japanese researchers, commented, "There is no proof the Indians and Dryden are being affected by the mercury." Another comment from Mr. Bernier: "There is no damage to the Indians of Grassy Narrows. The Canadian government will not act until the Canadian, and not the Japanese, verify the Indians are being harmed. I don't think we can rely on some traveling Japanese troubadours coming in and visiting these reserves on a one or two day basis and coming up with those kinds of findings."[24]

With that, Reed/Dryden, the company responsible for the Ojibway's exposure to mercury, continued to pollute, according to interviews in the news media with officials in Canada and the D'Itris, Smiths, and Lamms.[25] In 1974 Mr. Bernier had even asked Ottawa to raise the acceptable level of mercury in fish from 0.5 mcg/g, arguing, "Because Sweden and France accept a 1.0 ppm [level in fish] and Japan has no guidelines, we should look again at these levels imposed on us by the World Health Organization."[26] The reporter then asked Mr. Bernier, "So if you cannot reduce the mercury level in fish, you want to raise the acceptable standard of mercury?" "That's exactly right," he quickly answered. The journalist went on to report that Japan did have an acceptable standard—0.3 ppm (mcg/g)—and the standard in Sweden was stricter than Canada's, too.

The Canadian minister of the environment, George Kerr, did no better at showing that he was taking seriously the health of the Ojibway and the polluted fish problem. When asked in 1974 about keeping information of mercury poisoning a secret, he stumbled to find the right words: "There is no reason why any of these surveys which end up in a report, they shouldn't be made public; I think this is the only way to stop any rumors or erroneous statements about such analysis and report. So that this is a regular program of OWRC [Ontario Water Resources Commission] of examining various bodies of water. We've had one now for Clay Lake. This is available if anyone wants to look at it."[27]

The reporter commented, "The catch here is the phrase 'any of these surveys which ends up in a report.' If the Ministry has information, but hasn't put it in a report, then they say it's not for release, or they don't know where the data is, or it's not finished yet." Another yet to be publicly released government study, from 1973, stated, "The free flow of information and data on mercury in the environment with the problems of Ontario is impeded, for reasons that are not clearly understood."[28]

While these arguments were going on, the Ojibway continued to suffer. Fish intake was reduced on average but not for the guides. The sportfishing tourist industry was allowed to continue, despite the contamination. Even on Lake St. Clair, because Dow said it would reduce mercury dumping, fishing was reopened despite the continuing high levels of mercury in the lake's fish. One Ojibway guide stated, "The guides were expected to eat fish for lunch every day with the tourist guests. If they didn't, those tourists and their dollars might be frightened away and the guides would lose their jobs." This guide had a blood mercury level of 350 mcg/l, seventy times the EPA's ceiling of acceptability.[29]

Despite the Minamata diagnoses by Dr. Harada, and the fact that some of the Indians' mercury levels were even higher than some of those of Minamata, Leo Bernier still would say in 1975 of the Ojibway health tests, "There's nothing there that shows any degree of alarm." At one point in a CBC broadcast he announced that he was concerned with doing everything he could to "get these fish on the market." He suggested breading the fish so that by weight, with the bread, the level of mercury in the resulting "fish" would be reduced to less than 0.5 mcg/g.[30]

Finally, that year the Ontario Ministry of Health admitted there was a problem, and an alternative fish was distributed to the Indians, a fish that allegedly met the standards for mercury. Minister of Health F. S. Miller then concluded, "The medical people giving us the advice did not feel that people were exhibiting the symptoms of the disease and they were believed. Doctors have had trouble recognizing the problem."[31] It appears that their own government and the industry's doctors were the one's convincing the Canadians there was no problem. Their prejudice against the Japanese team blinded them further.

The following year, in a 1976 "interim report," toxicologist and Dow resin developer Thomas Clarkson released his findings. The highest recorded blood level in his testing of the people was 330 mcg/l. Of eleven guides tested, all had blood levels above 20 mcg/l, with a mean of 136 mcg/l.[32] Certainly, Dow managers then knew they had a problem, as their man, Clarkson, showed them the numbers. Perhaps the next question would be, did they accept that they had a problem? A published paper in 1979 by the Canadian Medical Services Branch, Health and Welfare Canada, and Clarkson disclosed that levels of mercury were taken from 356 communities and totaled 34,810 tests. Of these, 31 percent (10,822 people) had levels greater than 20 mcg/l, 740 individuals had levels greater than 100 mcg/l, and 61 had levels greater than 200 mcg/l. But, instead of reporting on an array of individuals and what the effects of high mercury levels had led to, the authors instead focused on just one individual. They stated that the purpose of their paper was simply to "focus on some of the problems involved in establishing the diagnosis of methylmercury poisoning in Canadian Indians."[33]

The authors of the report described only the case of a seventy-nine-year-old Cree Indian with a measured blood mercury level in 1975 of 551 mcg/l. On his physical exam in 1975, it was noted that he had tremor, diminished hearing, leg edema with sores on his legs, poor dental health, cardiac murmur, atherosclerosis, chronic lung disease, an enlarged heart, and sensory neuropathy as measured by an electromyogram. In the same year, he had an independent neurology consult that showed many abnormalities, including ataxia, diminished reflexes, and impaired mechanical performance tests when compared to his age group; he had a degree of neurological involvement entirely compatible with definite signs of chronic mercury intoxication, the neurologist concluded.

This individual succumbed to his disease two years later, and an autopsy was performed. The paper by the Canadian government, Wheatly, and Clarkson stated that his autopsy had been delayed and that he had "faulty preservation." It was concluded that the cause of death was aspiration pneumonia (caused by food getting into the lungs). After some further discussion, the paper's authors concluded, "Despite adequate knowledge of blood and hair levels over a three year period, plus clinical examinations, autopsy, extensive analysis of brain and tissue mercury levels, and neurohistology, a definitive diagnosis remains elusive in the present case."[34]

Elusive? This was certainly surprising to me when I read the case report and the literature available at the time. The researchers knew in 1979 that levels this high could be associated with the objective findings seen in this patient. This patient clearly had neurological symptoms consistent with mercury toxicity, and an independent neurologist had said as much. If the patient's neurological systems had been intact, perhaps he would have been able to swallow his food without inhaling it, preventing aspiration pneumonia and subsequent death.

The authors, it seems, did not want to come out and say he was affected by mercury. They were also silent on why researchers and government officials were having problems establishing a mercury diagnosis on the hundreds of other people who did not have any other disease during the investigation and were suffering from the effects associated with mercury toxicity.

In diagnostic medicine, many of our diagnoses are described using phrases such as "consistent with" and usually avoid the term "proven," as so many diseases overlap in their symptom profiles. The authors of the paper in question did not use the term "consistent with" or other similar terms in relation to effects of mercury toxicity. In this, their conclusions were not consistent with their findings. It seemed to be an exercise in how to avoid a lawsuit.

It was not so much the mercury load of the Cree man but the lower-exposure "symptoms" of mercury poisoning and the levels at which they could appear that constituted the "elusive" problem. Certainly, if industry had to compensate people for the symptom of fatigue, large numbers of individuals would qualify for compensation, as this was such a nonspecific complaint. The human mercury literature of the 1970s through the 1980s consisted of reports on accidental poisonings. The researchers did not have control groups, and sometimes not even an accurate mercury level in the study subject. They looked for overt symptoms that would be most specific to the disease. This was so they could be more certain of the diagnosis. Bias could enter at any point in the survey or study, as many researchers could have a conflict of interest if they took salaries, benefits, or grants from the industry whose polluting effects they were studying. Cases of poisoning, for which background evidence is often the results of epidemiologic studies that correlate varying degrees of exposure with symptoms, also pose the threat of courtrooms and lawyers if negligence or nuisance can be shown. This threat can add bias, as well, if the researchers feel threatened or encouraged in any way.

More or less coincident with the discovery of Canada's mercury contamination, the United States also reported results of elevated mercury concentrations in many of the nation's waterways. In the Philip Hart Senate Subcommittee hearings (Energy, Natural Resources, and the Environment), which began in May 1970 to discuss mercury contamination, numerous U.S. states reported incidents of mercury contamination.

Governor George Wallace of Alabama even called on the federal government to declare his state a disaster area. Commercial, noncommercial, ocean, and freshwater fish were being found to be mercury contaminated. This led to FDA and independent testing of canned tuna. The FDA sampling indicated that 23 percent, or 207 million of 900 million cans of tuna packed in 1970 had levels of mercury above 0.5 mcg/g, the standard even of the FDA at the time. The FDA commissioner then, Charles C. Edwards, declared that the fish were absolutely safe to eat—at the same time that he ordered them withdrawn from the market.[35]

By May 1971, the FDA reported that only 1 percent to 2 percent of canned tuna had mercury levels above 0.5 mcg/g. This was because it was discovered that two species of the fish, big-eyed tuna and yellowfin, accounted for most of the high numbers and were removed from the final report. The product codes for cans of those two species of tuna were then publicized for the purpose of a canned targeted tuna recall, with an alleged loss to the tuna industry of $84 million. It was this recall that prompted my mother to remove cans of tuna from her shelves.[36]

It had also been discovered that swordfish were over 0.5 mcg/g in mercury content 89 percent of the time. Swordfish consumers began coming forward with symptoms such as lethargy, frequent headaches, blurred vision, trembling hands, insomnia, loss of alertness, anxiety, and a feeling of "coming down with something." The symptoms disappeared after changing the diet. In May 1971, the FDA advised Americans to stop eating this fish altogether.[37]

This discussion of swordfish, which I first came across in 2004 in the D'Itri book, was just what I was looking for. If people did have symptoms of ill feeling from eating this type of fish, why did it not continue to be reported? Furthermore, the symptom profile matched the one for my patients. In fact, many people in the United States consume large predators such as swordfish and tuna regularly. That so little was said about the problem of mercury in fish suggested that politics and economic interests stood in the way of the dissemination of scientific knowledge.[38]

When it was discovered that many U.S. waterways were polluted by industry, the involved parties first had to look at what laws were being broken. Arguments ensued over which part of government was responsible and what laws or regulations were violated—or allowed the mercury to be dumped. Many acts of water quality and control had been passed by Congress over the years, but the laws were not being enforced. People of many states urged action from the federal government to force the polluters to stop dumping and provide money for cleanup. Hearings began to take place in 1970 out of concern for the environment and the economy. In one hearing, a member of the Hart Subcommittee asked Dr. Albert C. Kolbye Jr. of the FDA if he thought eating fish with 0.5 mcg/g of mercury was safe. Kolbye replied, "I would prefer to state that eating fish with 0.5 mcg/g levels of mercury certainly is far safer than eating fish with a higher level of mercury." As the D'Itris point out, by April of 1972, as the agency was trying to "reassure the public that a little poison was alright," the FDA reduced itself to using the analogy that a shot glass full of vermouth in a freight car full of gin was equivalent to a 0.5 mcg/g level of mercury in fish.[39]

Hundreds of lawsuits were filed in more than twenty states against mercury polluters in the 1970s. The Bass Anglers Society was especially active and filed more than two hundred suits in Alabama alone. The anglers also sued the secretary of the army and the Alabama Water Improvement Commission and called on the U.S. Army Corps of Engineers to set standards for refuse dumping. Much confusion arose when it turned out that the industries doing the polluting, such as many types of chemical plants, cement factories, and paper and pulp mills, did not know what was in their wastewater. Testing was not commonly done at the time, and testing capabilities were limited. In 1973, there were 2,668 major industrial dischargers in the United States located on 267 water basins. The water quality was below acceptable standards in 89 of those basins. Hearings would be ongoing to propose standards for waste discharges. In the end, the EPA announced that although almost all companies in the country could be prosecuted for previous illegal discharges, lawsuits would not be initiated if they applied for permits. As the D'Itris put it, "Forgive and forget." Compromises for some polluters would also be negotiated. Veils of secrecy were evident, as the U.S. government was reluctant to release the names of the polluters. Therefore, it is difficult to discover the human toll caused by the pollution.[40] Even today, many anglers do not know, do not understand, or do not care about the advisories given for the water they fish in.

In Canada in the 1970s, the mercury pollution situation became known as the "first mercury scare." Losses to the Canadian fishing and tourist industries, and the tuna and swordfish industries, as a result of the related U.S. "mercury scare" at the time ended up in the hundreds of millions of dollars. Court battles and negotiations were still ongoing in 2008, making it difficult to obtain information, especially directly from the Ojibway, as their leader did not answer my e-mails and researchers involved were unable to speak about the ongoing situation. The criteria by which the Canadian government assessed whether anyone was suffering from methylmercury poisoning were also not readily accessible. Thankfully, Dr. Harada returned in 2002 to reevaluate fifty-seven of the Indians in Whitedog and Grassy Narrows, where Dryden had dumped mercury into the waterway.

A unique aspect of Harada's report, published in 2005, was his description of the standard criteria used in Japan for diagnosis of Minamata disease. This is the only place I have found it in the English literature. First, a patient had to have sensory impairment of the extremities and around the mouth and one or more of the following: motor ataxia (difficulty with movement of the limbs), tunnel vision, impaired hearing, difficulty standing up, disturbed gait, disturbed ocular movement, tremor, and impaired speech. Harada went on to say that through Canada's Mercury Disability Board, set up in 1986, twenty-one victims who satisfied Minamata diagnostic criteria received $250–$800 (Canadian) per month. Thirteen did not file claims. About twenty of the fifty-seven individuals examined by Harada who met the criteria were denied compensation. Harada's report also noted that in his current investigation, as well as his investigation of 1975, there was a high rate of subjective and neurological symptoms. The most common subjective symptoms he noted were numbness, pain in the extremities, leg cramps, dizziness, headache, trembling, and forgetfulness. A significant factor that caught my eye was that the people observed still had elevated mercury levels in their hair in a range of from 0.11 to 18.0 mcg/g. The mean of the more severely affected group was approximately 3.5 mcg/g.[41] This meant that they were still actively exposed to mercury.

Difficulties surrounding the issue of mercury therefore continue for the Canadian Indians. The polluting industry and many scientists can say that the Indians' symptoms had other causes. One could also say that their symptoms are the lingering effects of their exposure in the 1970s. Then there is the possibility that they not only were affected by their past high exposure in the 1970s but are still being exposed and have not eliminated the source of their illness. In other words, if any of their symptoms are from current lower-level exposure, the failure to correct it all these years would have perpetuated their illness. Then there is the argument that telling the Indians not to eat fish would cause a devastating blow to their subsistence lifestyle—as some individuals with other interests would say, a little poisoning of the Indians doesn't mean you can't sell the fish to someone else. I think suffering from the various symptoms described would also be a severe blow to one's lifestyle. Perhaps the real issue is with the fishing industry, as they claim that people do not have adverse effects from methylmercury at these levels. My patients were able to obtain these mercury levels easily by consuming commercial fish. They had these symptoms, as well. They got better when they changed their diet and lowered their mercury levels.

Methylmercury discussions with the World Health Organization (WHO) have been ongoing over the last three decades. Back in 1990, WHO met to discuss the environmental health criteria for methylmercury. The resulting report (the first two drafts of which were prepared by Thomas Clarkson) discussed mostly the overt symptoms of methylmercury poisoning—those associated with neurological damage in general. The report stated that methylmercury poisoning was limited to the neurological system. Of course, the WHO also said that in an experiment in which pigs were given an oral lethal dose of methylmercury, death was preceded by diarrhea and vomiting. Further experimentation showed that in rats and dogs, anorexia preceded the clinical signs of nervous system injury. Other rodent experiments showed impairment of adrenal, testicular function, primary and secondary immune responses, sleep patterns, and thyroid function when the animals were given long-term doses. Perhaps they had a headache, fatigue, and muscle and joint pain, too, but how would anyone know? It is a known fact that rats can't vomit. Researchers rely on animal experimentation to assess chemical safety for humans. But using animals in this case may not tell us what we need to know. As we will find out later, though, the rats will have their day in court. As for humans, WHO relied heavily on data from Japan and Iraq and concluded that the nervous system was the principal target for the effects of methylmercury in adults—that the earliest effects were nonspecific symptoms of paresthesia, malaise, and blurred vision, and that damage was almost exclusively limited to the nervous system.[42] I certainly would want to find earlier warning signs of impending damage or doom in my patients.

Today, the Ojibway community still struggles. They lost their traditions when they could no longer fish as they had before and lost their health and well-being when poisoned. It was not until November of 1985 that a settlement was reached between the Canadian federal and the Ontario provincial governments: They would pay $5 million in compensation to the tribe and $2 million to set up a health fund. The Mercury Disability Board, mentioned in Harada's report, was set up to run the Health Fund program in the following year. Unfortunately, Indians were compensated only for medical expenses and lost income, and they were placed on welfare. They tried to grow rice on their land, but because of the construction of hydroelectric dams, their fields were flooded.

As for Chemical Valley, the pollution by other substances identified as endocrine disrupters was more recently implicated in shifts in the birth sex ratio and other health effects of the Aamjiwnaang First Nation community, members of the Ojibway tribe. From 1994 to 2003, a significant steady decline in the percentage of boys being born was evident, from 54 percent males to 35 percent males. The Ontario Ministry of the Environment and Energy knew in 1996 that multiple chemicals were polluting the Aamjiwnaang's reserve, and that these chemicals exceeded the government guidelines. So much for "water quality" agreements.[43]

So what happened to the lawsuit between Ontario province and

Dow that was filed in 1971? In a CBC radio interview in 1974 Dow was asked what was being done about the situation and gave this response: "There are a number of complicated legal issues and exceedingly complex facts in areas of new and rapidly evolving technology involved in the case."[44] Other reports suggested that when Dow stopped polluting, the mercury levels in the St. Clair went down, which made possible the reopening of fishing there in 1970. It was still unclear whether Dow dredged the area after the mercury scare, but in 1985, downstream from Dow's plant in Sarnia a large collection of toxic waste was discovered at the bottom of Lake St. Clair. It became known as the "Dow blob." The company vacuumed it up in 1985, but contamination in the lake attributed to Dow was still present. In 2002 and 2003, Dow began dredging again, in order to further clean up the contamination of previous years. Whether the blob was responsible for any deleterious human effects remains to be determined.[45]

All told, it appears that Dow and other polluting companies were able to get by with limited cleanups and compensation and could extend their court battles for many years. Industries such as Chisso in Japan and Dow and Reed/Dryden in Canada somehow found an acceptable level of mercury contamination to promote to the public as a level considered "safe" for human consumption. They could then admit that they contaminated the lake, but not enough to cause the harm that people were claiming. Therefore—so went the logic—their pollution was causing no harm, and they did not have to clean it up or compensate anyone. Above a certain mercury exposure level, you might have symptoms, and above another level you might have damage. Below a certain level, your symptoms were not from their contamination.

The waters were not only polluted, they became muddied as well. The United States and Canada could not simply say no one was affected. They had to have other evidence to counter the health claims people were beginning to make. That evidence began to become available in 1971, when Iraq suffered a methylmercury poisoning involving grain. The Iraqi incident would become the ticket out of court for industry, and it would become the leverage needed to force government agencies to loosen their regulations.

CHAPTER 10

Dr. Sa'adoun al-Tikriti

B ECAUSE MERCURY HAS BEEN INTRIGUING humans for centuries, it was surprising to me that the mercury-related advice coming from multiple agencies was so inconsistent. This left me and my patients in a state of bewilderment. The FDA Web site identified methylmercury poisoning symptoms—those my patients complained of. But the level of mercury in the blood at which those symptoms occurred was not in the report. Had adequate, careful studies been done? If so, by whom and on what populations? It seemed that too many of the papers on methylmercury in fish were interested in selling a product—fish. This seemed evident in the language of the discussion section at the end of a number of scientific papers. If members of the fishing industry encouraged hearty consumption of their product with a claim that it had medicinal value, they risk sounding like snake-oil salesmen or charlatans. (Curiously, some snakes have omega-3 fatty acids in their flesh, as well.)[1]

It is easy to sell a product to the public that is clean, is without toxicants, and has some sort of nutritional value. Having a contaminant present certainly gets in the way of profit. The problem is that many of the research papers pertaining to fish consumption and health do not tell us the contaminant levels in the fish the study subjects consumed, nor the type of fish, nor the omega-3 fatty acid content that is thought to be the key nutritional ingredient. Common sense would tell us that uncontaminated fish would be a better protein source than contaminated ones. But at what point the risk of contaminants outweighs the benefits of good nutrients is still being argued.

The FDA had taken the stance that there was a mercury level where deleterious effects on health began to occur, and if you had symptoms under that threshold, they just couldn't be from mercury. This level was not spelled out on the agency's Web site and was vague at best. Two hundred mcg/l for blood was that level, quoted to me by the California Public Health Department, but it took me considerable time and effort to confirm that it actually was the FDA's recommendation. The FDA wouldn't commit to telling the public that that was the level below which the agency believed a person would be without effects from methylmercury. In a teleconference, I was able to ask FDA officials whether they were going to review the literature and address the fact that adverse effects in humans began to occur at levels lower than 200 mcg/l in a number of instances.[2] They said it was not their responsibility to keep up with the literature; they had a committee looking into it. The Faroes childhood development study, the cardiac literature, symptom profiles in Japan, and infertility studies—all showing effects at levels less than 50 mcg/l—were, I guess, not being considered seriously by the FDA at the time. The fact that the entire spectrum of mercury effects on humans was still not clearly delineated posed a problem for the regulators as well as those exposed. To me, that meant my patients and I were on our own.

The policies that were in place for protecting the consumer, such as the levels of mercury allowed in fish in order for it to be fit for sale, were not enforceable. For the most part, it would be impossible and impractical even in 2008 to test every fish that came to the market. The FDA's limit of mercury in fish destined for commercial sale was 1 mcg/g. As the media and nongovernment organizations began testing on their own, they found that a significant number of large fish, and not just swordfish, exceeded that limit.

Modern mercury poisonings began about fifty years ago in multiple countries. Sweden, Pakistan, Guatemala, Japan, Canada, the United States, and Iraq all had human mercury poisonings between the late 1950s and the 1970s. Even so, good data that would be useful for a clinician was lacking.[3]

The fur hat industry, Japan's Chisso and Showa Denko plants, coal-fired power plants, the fishing industry, chlor-alkali plants, mercurial medicine, and vaccine makers, and even latex paint manufacturers (until 1991)[4] are just a small number of the industries that went through the process of neglect, deny, bury, and forget with respect to mercury. Most of the poisonings and health effects on humans were therefore evaluated within the winds of lawsuits, compensation to individuals, cleanup costs for the environment, the economy of the business or even the nation, and regulatory processes. But from compensation to cleanup, from U.S. Senate hearings to lawsuits, nothing was more confusing than the "scientific" literature itself when it came to the effects of mercury. Obviously, there was a discrepancy in the amount of mercury different agencies—the FDA and the EPA, particularly—thought was safe for humans. How that discrepancy came about and what was really at stake in the argument would be important to find out.[5]

Of immediate interest to me was how the California Public Health Department and allegedly the FDA had come up with a toxic threshold of 200 mcg/l in a person's blood, while the EPA said we should keep methylmercury in our blood at a level forty times lower, at less than 5.0 mcg/l, to be safe. It turned out to be a surprising and disturbing tale, indeed.

The California Public Health Department was the first to tell me that the standards set by the FDA were based on a poisoning that occurred in Iraq. This poisoning happened in the 1970s when a methylmercury fungicide was placed on grain intended not for direct consumption but for planting and sent to Iraq. People unwittingly ate the grain and became poisoned from the mercury. Studies subsequently were done, and the researchers involved concluded that an adult would be without negative health effects from mercury at levels up to 200 mcg/l. After this level paresthesias (numbness and tingling in the hands, feet, face, or other parts of the body) could be felt and could be the point at which permanent nerve damage began to occur. I was seeing an array of nonspecific symptoms in my patients at much lower levels of exposure, however.

One of the first papers written on this poisoning, an article published in 1973 in the journal *Science*, turned out to be one of the most useful. The fine print at the end explained that the observations on clinical symptoms were made by a list of Iraqis, and that the "data on hospital admissions were supplied by Dr. S. Tikriti, Directorate of Preventive Medicine, Ministry of Health, Iraq." Dr. Thomas Clarkson of the University of Rochester and Dow Chemical Company also was involved in the study of this poisoned population: He was listed as an author, and Dow Chemical was listed in the acknowledgments for providing its resin to be used on the Iraqis.[6]

The first time I read the paper, in 2000, the significance of the acknowledgments and where the poisoning took place did not register in my mind. But by 2004, I had been following the events in Iraq and the issues surrounding the Middle East, trying to understand why the U.S. military was there in the first place. It was in the doctors' dining room of the California Pacific Medical Center that I was able to get a feel for the emotions of this war-torn region. I just happened to be having lunch at the same table as a respected colleague who not only was from Iraq, but still went there every few months to visit family.

My Iraqi colleague was about my age, somewhere in his forties, and was always kind, thoughtful, and willing to help. When I explained what I had learned about the poisoning that took place in his country in 1971–1972, he told me he had not heard much about it. He continued to eat while I explained that the Iraqis and a researcher at the University of Rochester had studied the poisoning. When I mentioned that all the hospital data was provided by a Dr. S. Tikriti, though, he stopped and looked up at me, declaring, "Don't trust him." I asked if he knew him, and he said, "You meet one Tikriti, you've met them all. They are all crooks. They are all Saddam's men. Don't trust him."

Although it was clear that my colleague harbored a prejudice toward all Tikritis, he and another colleague helped me find a person who could tell me more about the Iraq incident and lead me to him.

Within a week, Dr. Dawood al-Thamery, a physician from Iraq who was visiting his daughter in California, came to see me. Dr. Thamery was a distinguished-looking, mustached man with gray hair, in his sixties, with a bright smile and dressed in a business suit. His wife, Muna al-Taha, a professor in Iraq, who was outspoken and well educated, accompanied him, as did their daughter. As we sat and had tea, it was clear that they were proud people and eager to defend their country from American misconceptions. Dr. Thamery did not like the American occupation, and he described the chaos that his country was currently in. He let me know that he and his wife had a good marriage, and that one was Sunni and the other Shiite. At one point, he got his business card out and started to hand it to me. It was from Saddam University. "Oh, wait," he said, crossing out Saddam's name and writing in the new name of the university. "Saddam ruined the Ba'ath party," he said tersely as he did so. Of course Dr. Thamery was a Ba'athi and seemed proud to tell me so.[7]

I tried to ask blunt questions about the events surrounding the poisoning. He was occasionally defensive, but he and his wife remained cordial. Dr. Thamery was a pediatrician at the time of the poisoning and had studied medicine at a top institution in the United States. He had "buried over 200 children alone" in the Iraq methylmercury seed grain disaster, he said sadly. He asked how many were reported dead. "According to the literature out of Iraq in the 1973 paper, 459," I replied. In fact, he quickly responded, no less than 4,000 had died. He explained that the hospitals had mostly the terminal cases; people came there to die, and few among the sick who would survive came in.

I asked about a statement in the 1973 article claiming that at blood mercury levels of less than 100 mcg/l, symptoms were from other causes. He said, "I do not believe this statement. They had no epidemiologic study. They did not go beyond the hospital [in Baghdad]." I asked if he would rely on this study to tell him and his daughters what a safe level of mercury was to consume while pregnant. He quickly replied, "No way." He said that "the Americans [the Rochester team] came with their resin," which did not work and had been administered too late to be effective, anyway.

"The Iraq poisoning was a blow to the Iraqi government, and you do not want to embarrass the government," Dr. Thamery went on. I asked if he thought people were afraid or inhibited in any way from coming forward when they were ill, and he claimed not. He then explained, "I had no problem with Saddam. I could criticize . . . well, I never criticized him at a personal level, but I could speak out within my jurisdiction." What relationship had Dr. Tikriti with Saddam? Dr. Thamery didn't answer directly but said, "Oh, the name Tikriti does not mean he is a relative, just that he was from Tikrit." I said, "I understand, but he also goes by Sa'adoun. Isn't the Sa'adoun tribe the most loyal to Saddam?" He said, "Well, yes." He later told me that Saddam had given Sa'adoun money and support for Sa'adoun's child, who was dying of cancer. He changed the subject and remarked of the fallen leader, "Saddam wanted his name and picture everywhere so that a thousand years from now they would think he was a great ruler of importance."

It was not until the end of our visit that Dr. Thamery let on that he knew Sa'adoun well. He was almost on his way out the door when he said, "Here, I will give you his phone number."

So now we had three levels of mercury in the body that were said to have some sort of significance. Below 5 mcg/l was what the EPA believed safe; below 100 mcg/l the symptoms should be attributed to something other than mercury, according to the 1973 *Science* paper; and then there was the 200 mcg/l, allegedly from the FDA.

In the next week, I phoned Dr. Tikriti from my office. He clearly had been told I would be calling.[8] I told him I was interested in the 1971–1972 Iraq methylmercury poisoning and understood that he might be the one who held the answers. He said, "Perhaps I should come visit you, and we will meet and talk and I will answer all your questions." I felt then that I should not let him go—I might not get another chance. I said I just wanted to ask a few questions. "Well, okay, then," he replied.

Dr. Tikriti was friendly, with almost the same demeanor as Dr. Thamery. He had come to the United States the prior year, after the fall of Saddam, in 2003, and was retired. In Iraq he was the "director general," a position he likened to that of the U.S. surgeon general, and a professor of public health, at the University of Baghdad. "More than sixty thousand people were affected by the mercury poisoning," he said. He and a team of researchers from the University of Rochester did a retrospective study on the people using hair mercury analysis. When I asked about the details, he said that no formal questionnaire had been given to the study subjects and that they were only asked questions in person.

It appeared that Dr. Thamery may have been right, that from the Iraqis' perspective, there had not been a formal epidemiologic study conducted in this incident that could form the basis of solid policy decisions.

The most severely affected among the poisoned suffered from ataxia (gross incoordination of muscle movements), blindness, and death, Dr. Tikriti said. When I asked about the lower exposures and how mercury was seen to affect people, he replied, "Below 100 mcg/l you have minor symptoms such as headache, leg pain, fatigue, weakness, especially if long time exposure. If the exposure continued, there could be permanent damage." Would he rely on the studies from Iraq to tell his daughters how much mercury was safe to consume? Like Dr. Thamery, he said, "No way." When asked if the incident was an accident, he quickly said, "It was my mistake that people got sick. I did not do a good enough job to warn them. It was all my fault. This was an embarrassment to my country. I will write a book about it." He then said, without any prompting, "Okay, I have a lot of data that was not given to the World Health Organization and was unpublished for political reasons. I am ready to speak, but I need time to prepare." I then tried to press him on whether he thought that the incident was an accident or that Saddam had a motive to purposefully poison certain populations. He cut me off, saying, "That is political. I cannot comment on that." At this point, he did not want to answer any more of my questions or go into more detail about the poisoning. Afterward, he did not answer my e-mails, either—perhaps because Saddam was still alive at the time.

Our conversation was strained at best, and I did not feel it was my place to interrogate him. Sa'adoun al-Tikriti was the man who "made a mistake" or was perhaps the fall guy. In any case, a massive poisoning of the people of Iraq had ensued. He did not give all the data to WHO for political reasons. He did not have any formal questionnaire to use as the basis for a uniform study, but studies were reported using the data he provided. His "mistake" was an embarrassment to his country, and many people suffered from the poisoning. Had he owed Saddam a favor, or was he just a loyal subject?

The Iraqi methylmercury seed grain poisoning became a disturbing puzzle I had not previously considered. If Dr. Tikriti did not turn over all the data and presumably was under political pressure to downplay the extensiveness of the poisoning's effects in the outcome of the study, the reliability of the data for any scientific application would be questionable. Many of my colleagues in the mercury world believed that it was the Americans who were "in charge" of the Iraqi studies, but what they did not consider was that the Iraqis controlled the number and type of data points that made it to the statistician's computer.

CHAPTER 11

Fishy Loaves

A T THIS POINT, one would still be confused as to how to assess patients when it came to methylmercury toxicity. How important was the Iraqi study for making policy around the world when it came to mercury in fish and judgments of mercury toxicity more generally? "The importance of the study in Iraq is that it is still used as the basis for the assessment of risk to human health by World Health Organization and regulatory agencies," WHO stated succinctly in a 2000 report. By 2004, WHO did urge caution in using the Iraqi data for such assessments, though, only because the number of study subjects was small and, well, bread may be different than fish.[1]

I felt compelled to investigate the Iraq situation, considering the information provided by the Iraqi's former minister of health Dr. Tikriti and the pediatrician Dr. Thamery, who witnessed the poisoning episode, as well as the subsequent U.S. involvement in Iraq. The Iraqi mercury incident that occurred in 1971–1972 turned out to be the largest and most bizarre mass mercury poisoning in history. It was not the first methylmercury poisoning in that country, though, and it began with a common practice in the treatment of grain not peculiar to that country.

In many countries where seed grain is imported and distributed by the thousands of tons, pests, molds, and fungi are a problem. It was discovered long ago that methylmercury, when used on seed grain, could effectively reduce the molds and fungi that cause a tremendous loss of crops. The makers of these fungicides claimed that if a farmer planted the mercury-laced grain and did not eat it directly, the resulting grain harvested for food would be safe. Many different mercury fungicides were made by multiple companies from the 1940s through the 1970s.

Unfortunately, there were numerous incidents in which people either were not able to, or simply did not, follow the directions for planting, resulting in mercury poisoning to humans, livestock, and wild animals. The best known of the historical outbreaks of human poisoning from seed grain laced with mercury fungicide occurred in Iraq in 1956 and 1960, Pakistan in 1961, and Guatemala in 1965. Sweden also discovered and made public that this type of fungicide was contaminating their people, wildlife, and foodstuffs and banned it in 1966. According to the D'Itris, the United States had halted the interstate trade of methylmercury seed grain in 1970, but unfortunately allowed companies in the United States to export methylmercury-fungicided grain to other nations for years afterward.[2]

A curiosity about accounts of the events surrounding the Iraq seed grain poisoning of 1971–1972 was that history books about Saddam's Iraq included no reference to the poisoning, at least that I could find. At the same time, the sparse scientific literature that was published about the poisoning did not discuss the political context in which it occurred. The Iraqi government itself, as one might expect, encouraged little independent investigation of the poisoning, its effects, or how it had been possible.

The first and still primary scientific report in a scientific publication, I found, was the article published in *Science* in July 1973, discussed in chapter 10. The authors indicated that the team of researchers investigating the poisoning only looked at individuals within a sixty-three-mile radius of Baghdad Hospital.[3] This confirmed the statement of Dr. Thamery that the researchers did not venture far from the Baghdad Hospital. Although the paper noted that 6,530 individuals presented at the hospital, only 125 were studied for symptomatology, and blood levels were not collected until at least several months after the poisoning began. According to Dr. Tikriti, an additional report prepared by WHO looked at information on almost 2,000 affected individuals, though the "data" on which it was based were, as with the other studies, all provided by Dr. Tikriti.[4]

Dr. Thamery and his wife and Dr. Tikriti had all told me that the Iraqi physicians at the time of the poisoning did not have the capabilities for conducting any large-scale epidemiologic study of the people affected, nor did they attempt one.

Frank and Patricia D'Itri discovered that the poisoned grain entered Iraq in the first place through a complicated trade agreement negotiated between the Iraqi government and Cargill Incorporated of Minneapolis, or one of its international subsidiaries, under which 73,202 metric tons of treated wheat and 22,262 metric tons of treated barley were imported.[5]

One of the few independent investigative reporters who documented this poisoning, Edward Hughes, writing in the *London Sunday Times*, suggests that successive droughts in 1969 and 1970 had devastated crop production and led the Iraqi government to import large quantities of grain. This all occurred, Hughes points out, not long after the Ba'ath party's 1968 coup d'état that brought that party to power.[6] Hughes's account gives the impression that he was suspicious about some aspect of the Iraqi's side of the story, and perhaps a bit angry. Now that the Ba'ath regime has fallen in Iraq, we may be able to learn more about this terrible disaster that occurred in 1971.

According to Hughes, the "authorities ordered" that farmers be provided with great quantities of foreign seed and, for reasons not transparent, purposely requested twice what was needed. For the bulk of the wheat seed, they chose Mexipak, a high-yield seed developed as part of the Green Revolution by American Nobel Prize winner Norman Borlaug at the Rockefeller Foundation's wheat improvement station in Mexico.

The bulk of the wheat order, 63,000 tons, came from Cargill. The head of Cargill's "oriental" division flew from his office in Geneva to Iraq to thank the Iraqis for the order, which he said was the largest wheat seed order in world history. Most of the wheat seed came from Mexico. According to a report to WHO by another Iraqi researcher, the 22,000 tons of barley came from suppliers in California.[7]

The Iraqi government requested that all the grain be treated with a mercury fungicide, the accounts of Hughes and of the scientific literature agree. And on September 16, 1971, the freighter SS *Trade Carrier* brought to Basra its deadly cargo.[8]

Cargill, founded in 1865 by W.W. Cargill, in Conover, Iowa, is one of the world's largest privately owned companies. Cargill initially began in the grain industry but quickly expanded to oil, steel, waste disposal, metal processing, plastics, animal feed (including fishmeal), beef, pork, poultry, salt, petroleum, coal—and the list goes on. With ConAgra, the company currently controls 50 percent of U.S. grain exports.[9] I was unsuccessful in my attempts to get anyone from the company to talk to me about the grain shipment to Iraq and its aftermath. When I asked about the incident, I was simply told that the company was privately owned and was referred to its Web sites.[10]

According to Hughes, years earlier, in 1956, several hundred Iraqi peasants had been poisoned by mercury-treated seed, and some had died. Had many officials not been shot or forced from their posts in the revolutionary purge of 1958, steps might have been taken by the Ministry of Health or Agriculture to prevent a repetition of the tragedy. But it was repeated. Another poisoning with the same type of fungicide occurred in 1960, injuring thousands and killing at least one hundred, according to Hughes. "Since dozens of officials who coped with that disaster were, in turn, swept away in the Ba'athists' slaughter of the Qassim regime in 1963," he tells us, "it was something of a miracle that any experts at all were left in 1971." These earlier Iraqi poisonings were reported in the scientific literature, it should be said, but not in the detail Hughes provided.[11]

The Iraq methylmercury seed grain poisoning of 1971–1972 and the Canadian and U.S. mercury scares coincided with the recommendations on mercury and fish consumption by the U.S. FDA and the Canadian government. As the authors of the 1973 paper in *Science* wrote, "The study of the population exposed to methylmercury that we describe in this article is of great importance." This was preceded by a lengthy discussion of how much the mercury issue had damaged the fishing industry, indicating that the information obtained in the Iraq poisoning would be ever so important. From the very beginning of this investigation, it appears that the researchers wanted to use the data collected in the poisoning to determine what amount of exposure caused harm and what the effects were. The clinical discussion of the poisoning in the *Science* paper concluded that at mercury concentrations of 1–100 mcg/l, symptoms were probably caused by factors other than mercury. No data, methods, or statistical proof of that statement were given.[12]

In my interview with Dr. Tikriti in 2004, he did not agree with these clinical conclusions of the authors of the 1973 article, and he was the one providing all the data to the researchers. He was also one of the article's authors. But then, he did not provide all the data he had, he admitted. He also never conducted a symptom survey or a true epidemiologic study. The "data" were hand picked by him. He told me, as mentioned in the preceding chapter, that at levels less than 100 mcg/l minor symptoms did occur, especially if the person was exposed to mercury for a long time.[13] This fact is extremely important to those who have continually made the claim that they were affected by mercury at much lower levels of exposure than reported in the literature, and gives some validation to what the Japanese researchers, the Canadian Indians, and my patients had been saying, as well.[14]

When I first read the 1973 *Science* paper, I was curious as to why the authors were interested in the fishing industry economy or the health of consumers of fish in a study of a land-based episode of mercury poisoning. It was not until I began looking into the historical aspects of mercury and health issues that I discovered what might be the answer. One of the authors of the *Science* paper was Thomas Clarkson of the University of Rochester, the same person who had also been in Canada making reports to the Canadian government about the effects of mercury-laden fish on the Ojibway and developing a resin that promised to eliminate mercury faster in the body, under the auspices of Dow.

As for the Iraqi scientists involved, some conflicts of interest existed during the time of the investigation into the poisoning. The Tikritis did have a reputation for supporting Saddam Hussein, as Saddam himself was a Tikriti. Also, I later found out, the lead author of the 1973 paper, Dr. Farhan Bakir, claimed to be Saddam's personal physician, a claim that Dr. Thamery confirmed.[15]

When the grain poisoning was discovered, the Iraqis initially invited the world's scientists to help them by sending out an inconspicuous distress call in a letter to the *British Medical Journal* in March 1972. "We would like to draw attention to an outbreak of poisoning from the mercurial compound Granosan M, which has ravaged Iraq in the last two months," it read. "A similar outbreak on a smaller scale occurred in this country in 1961 and has been reported. It will be greatly appreciated if doctors from other countries with experience in this field, particularly as regards treatment, would correspond with the undersigned."[16]

Granosan M, manufactured by DuPont, was allegedly the cause of the previous poisonings in Iraq, but the Rochester researchers did not report finding the Granosan compound, ethylmercury-p-toluenesulfonanilide, in their laboratory analysis of the 1971–1972 poisoning. The authors did say that the Iraqis may have added additional fungicides, including the Granosan M compound, locally. Because of the enormous size of the grain order that was the source of the poisoning, multiple companies may have contributed seed to the project and used a variety of mercury compounds to treat it. Panogen was one fungicide used, for example, according to Edward Hughes, and he photographed one of its bags for the *London Sunday Times*.[17]

In 1972, Clarkson of the University of Rochester and Hamish Small of Dow Chemical responded to the Iraqis' distress call. Why Dow? Dow would have been interested not only in how its resin did, but also in the opportunity to obtain information that could protect the company's interests back home. Dow was facing a $35 million lawsuit, filed in March 1971 by the province of Ontario for consequences of the company's mercury pollution. Dow was also threatened with a lawsuit by the State of Ohio for polluting the waterways with mercury. It was certainly convenient for Dow to have one of its researchers in Iraq participating in the study of the poisoned subjects and taking advantage of an opportunity to direct the analysis of any health effects of methylmercury that were evident.[18]

Clarkson arrived in Iraq with neatly packaged doses of his Dow resin—for two hundred mice or two humans, though it had not yet been tested in humans. The Dow Chemical Company rushed one hundred pounds of the resin to Iraq after obtaining emergency approval by the FDA for its use, only to find it was too late for it to be of benefit to the already ill and dying people. The Iraqi physicians were asked to administer it anyway, and Clarkson and his colleagues then wrote papers about how it reduced the half-life of mercury in the human body. Perhaps the reason no one heard much about this resin is that Clarkson discovered that sodium 2,3-dimercaptopropane-1-sulfonate (DMPS) was more effective.[19] Was this, then, the new and rapidly evolving technology that Dow spoke of in 1974 that had delayed court proceedings between Dow and the Ontario government? In any case, the resin, if it had proven effective, would certainly have been a wonder drug that would have helped Dow Chemical and other polluters and the fishing industry.[20]

Why the Iraqis, who had more experience with poisoning from this type of fungicide than anyone in the world, would order nearly 100,000 tons of the fungicide-treated grain and not issue a caution as to its use may remain a mystery.

Saddam and his government knew the circumstances that could lead to the improper use and subsequent death of the consumer when it came to methylmercury-fungicided grain. They were also surely aware that their countrymen and people of other nations had properly used this fungicide without known ill effects. Previous papers published about the smaller-scale mercury fungicide poisoning in Iraq of 1960 were done with incredible detail. The Iraqi scientists also wrote in 1960, "[Mercury poisoning] is as old as the Roman Civilization when mercurialism was known as the disease of slaves."[21] Some Iraqi authors who wrote papers in peer-reviewed journals on the previous poisonings and who were well versed in the history of mercury were still active in their native country and, in fact, were among the authors of the *Science* article on the 1971–1972 poisoning, so there was no lack of knowledge or expertise to draw on if the government chose to do so.

Whether this 1971 poisoning was an accident or had malicious intent was important to discuss, as it was used to set the standards for allowable mercury in humans and fish, and to assess methylmercury toxicity effects in humans for years to come. Certainly, Tikriti's hand-picking of the data and limiting the Rochester researchers' access to patients and information during the process of data collecting would lend question to the validity of the papers that were subsequently published. This would reveal a potential bias that had previously not been considered by the scientific community or WHO.

How and why had that poisoning in 1971–1972 taken place, I wondered. Mercury and environmental scientists often quote various scientific papers that came out of that poisoning episode, seemingly taking everything at face value, regardless of whether they agree with the findings and conclusions. With the additional insight gained from speaking to the Iraqi physicians, I felt it necessary to look deeper into the situation. If the world's mercury assessments have been hanging on the gallows of Saddam's regime, then we should all know about it.

In reading the history books on Iraq and Saddam, two facts came up over and over again. First, public insult to the president, or of the top institutions of the state or party, was punishable by life of imprisonment or death, which meant there was unlikely to be critical literature on the poisoning. And second, Saddam was notorious for being utterly ruthless when it came to perceived enemies. Saddam's first assassination, after all, was of his brother-in-law, also named Sa'adoun al-Tikriti. Whether he was any relation to Dr. Sa'adoun al-Tikriti of the Ministries of Health is unknown at this time.[22] And Saddam was known for openly employing the Stalinist maxim "If there is a person, then there is a problem; if there is no person, then there is no problem."[23] It turned out as well that Saddam knew from his past a surprising amount about the agricultural countryside and, most likely, much about methylmercury seed grain.

Soon after the February 1963 coup that brought the Ba'ath party to power, according to historian and author Con Coughlin, Saddam was given a minor position at the Central Farmers' Office. His activities there were apparently not just agricultural, though:

> Apart from his mundane duties at the Central Farmers' Office, he [Saddam] became closely involved in organizing the National Guard, the brownshirts of the Ba'ath party. He visited detention camps in Baghdad and helped to supervise the "punishment" of communist detainees. Some of the detainees were held at the

peasant camp, which provides an intriguing insight into the likely nature of Saddam's duties at the Central Farmers' office. Saddam's task it appeared was to improve the lot of the peasants, so long as they were peasants who did not have communist sympathies.[24]

A news interview with one of Saddam's boyhood friends also indicates that Saddam worked in the Iraqi Ministry of Agriculture in the early to mid-1960s. This is important to know, as it increases the likelihood that he knew about and recognized the consequences of the grain poisoning that occurred in 1960.[25]

It is unclear how long Saddam remained in the farmers' office, but by summer of 1964 he had been promoted to the Ba'ath party's regional command. Soon thereafter he was incarcerated for conspiring against the country leadership, but in 1966 he escaped, though it has been commonly said that the guards simply let him walk out.[26]

After the Ba'ath party regained power in the July 1968 coup, Sunnis from Tikrit quickly began to dominate the government. Ahmad Hassan al-Bakr became president, and Saddam, a relative, the heir apparent. Saddam Hussein al-Tikriti, whose name means "one who confronts," became the undersecretary general of the Revolutionary Command Council (RCC) in January 1969; then a few months later, he became vice president.[27] As Saddam rose to power, he eliminated rivals and other opposition figures.[28]

Against that background it is easy to wonder whether there might have been some intention to poison or for the government to do less than it could to save lives once the grain was distributed. Then as now, Iraq was deeply divided along ethnic lines. Sunni Arabs, among them Hussein's family, constitute 20 percent of Iraq's population, and most live in the area north of Baghdad between the Tigris and Euphrates Rivers. In the fertile, densely inhabited river plain south of Baghdad the majority of Shiites reside and constitute about 55 percent of the population. The Kurds are non-Arab, mostly Sunni people, who live mainly in the mountains of northern Iraq. They make up 15 percent to 20 percent of the population, and in the early 1970s one of their strongholds was the heartland of Iraq's oil fields in Kirkuk.[29]

According to the 1973 *Science* paper, the grain was dispensed to all provinces of the country, but more than 50 percent of the total distribution went to the three northern provinces of Nineveh, Kirkuk, and Arbil. The grain was delivered to local granaries throughout the country, which, in turn, distributed it to the farmers. Given the numbers cited in the article, 78 percent of the total distributed wheat grain and 74 percent of the total distributed barley went to the then Kurdish majority areas of Nineveh, Kirkuk, Arbil, Diyala, Sulaimaniya, and D'hok.[30]

A paper written by five Iraqi scientists, including Saddam's physician, F. Bakir, and printed in the *World Health Bulletin* gave similar statistics and detailed where the barley was distributed, though not the wheat. Barley was mainly used for the animals, whereas the wheat was used for humans.[31]

Edward Hughes may be right that not much was done to prevent or ameliorate the poisoning in part because many agricultural and poison experts who could have helped may already have been eliminated for political reasons. But Saddam himself, if he knew of the grain distribution, would have known of its implications and could have done more to prevent the disaster. He not only worked in the Farmers' Office shortly after poisonings in the past, but also was in charge of the ministries and may even have been the one to give the order to purchase such a large amount of grain. It is difficult to believe that the government simply had forgotten about the previous poisonings or thought that this type of fungicide would not cause harm the third time they ordered it.[32]

During the 1971–1972 poisoning, the incidence of mercury illness varied considerably by area. According to the 1973 *Science* paper, the researchers did not know the precise time at which the grain was given to the farmers, "but deliveries for some farmers may have continued into January 1972—the time when the authorities issued stringent warnings concerning the danger of consuming the grain."[33] The papers written by other Iraqi scientists said simply that the tainted seed was given to the farmers after they had planted their own grain. The warnings on the sacks themselves were written in Spanish and English. Some of the sacks had the skull and crossbones on them, but this meant nothing to the Iraqi culture at the time.

Hughes's accounts of what happened next are the most thorough, as he interviewed the people on the ground in Iraq:

> This time the fatal flaw lay in the very concept of the grain distribution scheme. Having ordered far more wheat than was needed, the authorities sought to curry favour with peasants by distributing it free of charge. Repayment in kind would await the next harvest many months away. When word of a free handout spread across the countryside, farmers rushed to sell their own wheat stocks before prices fell. With empty bins, they could justify a claim for more of the government's imported grain. But empty bins meant that such peasants would have to depend on the new Mexipak both for their seeding and for their baking oven all winter.[34]

The grain came too late for many farmers. Although it arrived in Basra in plenty of time for the October-November planting, getting it by truck to isolated farms, sometimes far to the north, was a problem. An official committee developed some safety plans, including use of a small plane to drop half a million warning leaflets among five million people on the land. Initially, the grain shipments were carefully guarded, but the officials abandoned the effort two weeks after they started. "Truck drivers were carefully trained to hurry their cargoes directly to distribution warehouses, yet some got lost, while others arrived with missing sacks, reporting that they had been robbed. As for the requirement that each farmer sign or put his thumbprint on a statement that he knew the grain he was receiving was poison, some distributing agents from the start dispensed with this as a troublesome bit of red tape," Hughes reports.[35]

So what did the people do with this free grain? Instead of planting it like they were supposed to, some, perhaps from ignorance, perhaps from desperation, ground it up and made bread out of it. The grain had been dyed pink to indicate the presence of mercury fungicide. Some people washed off the pink dye, thinking the grain could then be eaten. The problem was, the dye washed out, but the mercury did not. Some first fed it to their livestock for a few days; since the animals seemed to be fine, the farmers then ate the grain. The problem here was that mercury accumulates, and the effects of daily doses, whether for humans or other animals, took weeks and perhaps months to become evident. Subsequently, their livestock was seen to be contaminated and was banned from sale. Some farmers thought the pink dye was a government trick and the warnings could therefore be ignored.[36]

So, arrival after farmers had planted their own grain for the season, lack of warnings, people's need for economic survival, and hunger could all have contributed to people eating the allotment of grain instead of planting it. The number of people who could have been affected was enormous. It was estimated that a thousand tons of grain could poison sixty thousand people.

After several months, people began pouring in to the hospitals. But instead of spreading word to others of the harm in eating the contaminated grain, the government imposed a news blackout. Here is Hughes again: "The first warnings of a national epidemic had reached Iraqi authorities on December 26, 1971. At the main hospital in Kirkuk, Iraq's oil capital of the North, doctors suddenly had been deluged with peasants with advanced ataxia and paresthesias. 'Luckily,' one of the doctors at Kirkuk had attended patients in the 1960 poisoning crisis and immediately diagnosed the problem."[37]

According to Hughes, Dr. Sa'adoun al-Tikriti, director of preventive medicine at the ministry, flew with his aide to Kirkuk. Other cities also reported cases, and a scramble for what was then the only treatment, BAL—British anti-Lewisite—was being ordered in massive quantities.[38] Also known as dimercaprol, BAL was a very old agent that had been used for heavy metal poisonings since the 1940s. At the time, it was not known which agents would work for methylmercury poisoning; unfortunately, BAL was later determined not to be very effective.

Perhaps it was coincidental that Kirkuk was the first recognized area in which poisoning occurred on a large scale, or perhaps the government was most interested in what effects the poison was having on the people of that region. Regardless, here is where Thomas Clarkson came into play, because his resin might work better than BAL. Hughes reports, "A team from the University of Rochester was invited by Baghdad authorities to study the tragedy, headed by the eminent toxicologist

Dr. Thomas Clarkson. Rochester's mercury poisoning research unit is widely regarded as the world's best in its field." And: "Other Rochester data is helping science determine how much mercury men, women, and children can safely absorb in their diets."[39]

Clarkson did indeed conduct experiments on how a variety of agents affected people. In a paper published in 1981, he reported that he had given forty-seven patients affected from the Iraq seed grain poisoning different agents, including his Dow resin, two types of penicillamines, and sodium 2,3-dimercaptopropane-1-sulfonate (DMPS), to study the results of each. In the end, DMPS appeared to work best, as it accelerated the removal of mercury from the body by a factor of four, the Dow resin by a factor of three, and the penicillamines by about two. But then again, the Iraqis supplied all of the "analytical data." Dr. Tikriti, as he had told me, was in charge of providing the patients, blood samples, and subsequent mercury results for all the data that came out of Iraq, and subsequently, what this paper's conclusions and the conclusions of all other papers coming out of Iraq were based on.[40]

After the poisoning was well under way, the Iraqi government recalled the poisoned seed and decreed the death penalty for anyone selling it. People, frightened, dumped some of the seed into the Tigris River; as a consequence, the sale of local fish was also forbidden because of "potential poisoning." According to Hughes, the Iraqi government put out only "discrete little announcements in the newspaper and the radio about the poisoning." The D'Itris came to a similar conclusion: The government instituted a news blackout when the epidemic began, and only brief official announcements were released in the state-controlled newspapers and radio broadcasts.[41]

Unofficial estimates were that up to tens of thousands of people could have eaten enough to cause some damage to themselves. Tourists reported that thousands of people suffered brain damage, blindness, and paralysis.[42] While the government officially acknowledged initially that 6,530 victims were hospitalized and 459 died, both Dr. Tikriti and Dr. Thamery said that at least ten times that many were affected, and that the people who came to the hospital were mainly the ones who came there to die. Two areas that had among the highest concentrations of those affected, according to the authors in *Science*, were a predominantly Kurdish region of the north, Kirkuk, and a heavily Shiite area of the south, Muthanna.

When Hughes was able to tour parts of Iraq two years after the event, he came to this conclusion:

> My investigation and the private estimate of experts on the scene suggests that as many as 6,000 may have died, and perhaps 100,000 were injured. Most are left to limp along the back lanes of rural Iraq, or to huddle, twitching in the doorways of their mud huts. Among this debris can be counted the twisted children grotesquely playing football. On the sidelines was a ten-year-old boy who must be carried everywhere, his brother half walks, half crawls on two hands and one foot.[43]

In June 1972, an editorial in the *British Medical Journal*, noting the necessity of developing standards for acceptable daily intake of mercury, commented on the incident and its aftermath: "Unfortunately, the seed grain was dressed with a mercurial compound known to produce irreversible injury in man," and "the devastation in Iraq is probably less amenable to therapy and rehabilitation." The editorial went on, "There is danger that hypothetical hazards will attract study while little is done to prevent real hazards, for it is easier to form pious resolutions than to stop people doing dangerous things. But the manufacturers and distributors of substances known to be dangerous can be identified and their activities controlled—though probably only by the concerted action of medical men."[44]

Why did the Kurds, with just 15 percent to 20 percent of Iraq's population, receive this grain out of proportion to other groups in Iraq, I still wondered. Perhaps they were in more desperate need. Or they just planted more grain than any other group. I was unable to find specific information on the cultivation practices in Iraq by region for 1971–1972. Could there also have been a motive of Saddam's for "purging" the enemy at that particular time? Was there an enemy?

Iraq contains the world's second-largest oil reserves after Saudi Arabia. In 1971, control of the country's oil industry was vested in the Iraq

Petroleum Company (IPC), a consortium of five of the world's largest oil companies: BP, Shell, Esso, Mobil, and Compagnie Française des Pétroles (CFP). The IPC, which had been organized in part by Qassim, the previous leader of Iraq, accounted for the entire oil production of Iraq and effectively controlled prices and quotas. This was viewed as a kind of foreign occupation of the Iraqi economy, and the Ba'ath party was eager for the Iraqi government to gain ultimate control over the country's oil wealth.[45]

In 1971, Saddam, together with the oil minister, assumed responsibility for dealing with the oil consortium. To nationalize the IPC, Saddam first needed to form alliances. Although he was anti-communist, he was even more anti-imperialist. He felt that an alliance with the Soviets would give him access to arms purchases and, at the same time, Soviet protection from Iran. The Soviets said they would support nationalization of the IPC and purchase any Iraqi oil surpluses. Saddam also developed an alliance with the French government, which said it would decline to join a boycott for nationalizing the IPC so long as French interests were not harmed. "So long as we have oil, we have power," Saddam is said to have commented. "I want Iraq to have the last barrel of oil in the world."[46]

Before the nationalization of the IPC took place, battles for the oil-fields were ongoing. Both the Shiites in the south and the Kurds in the north were considered a problem for the Ba'ath. Despite this, Saddam began secret negotiations with the Kurdish leader Mustafa Barzani, and one text claims that Saddam personally directed attempts to accommodate the Kurds' wish for self-autonomy.[47] By March 1970, a fifteen-point deal was made known as the March Manifesto. Barzani wanted Kirkuk to be the capital of a Kurdish autonomous region, on the basis of its province having a Kurdish majority. Because Kirkuk was also the heartland of Iraq's oil fields, Saddam argued that the Kurds constituted a majority only in certain parts of Kirkuk and that only those areas with a majority should be included in the autonomous region.

The fifteen-point agreement, carefully planned by Saddam, provided a four-year period for the provisions of the agreement to take full effect—ample time for him to rearrange the demographic balance in

Kurdistan, Kirkuk especially, in his favor. In September 1971, some forty thousand Shiite Kurds were expelled to Iran on the grounds that they were not really Iraqis. And on the 29th of that month, just two weeks after the grain had come to Basra, an attempt was made on Barzani's life.[48]

I have yet to find a history book that mentions that the Iraqi seed grain poisoning occurred in the Kirkuk area at the same time Saddam was trying to gain control of the oil fields by altering the demographics of the area. Here is a proposition historians might consider: After being poisoned by a methylmercury-fungicided seed grain given to them by the Ba'ath regime, the Kurdish people were without bread, were not able to sell or eat much of their livestock because of the poison they had fed to their animals, and were not allowed to fish in the river because the fish were thought to be contaminated. Tens of thousands of Kurds of Iranian origin were forced out of Iraq in 1972 alone. Others too, left the region, as they were starving, dying, sickened, and, in some cases, maimed for life and feared worse events to come. This made room for the growing numbers of Iraqi Arabs arriving in the area of Kirkuk. Though the Ba'ath regime may not have intentionally poisoned the population (after all, distribution wasn't confined to the Kurds), it seems quite plausible that they found ways to take advantage of the poisoning and good reason to drag their heels in recalling the grain and treating its victims. On June 1, 1972, Saddam made his move and nationalized the IPC.

When the census of the Kurdish region was completed in March 1974, in accord with the March Manifesto, the government's autonomy plan was put into effect. Barzani rejected the agreement and said he wanted instead extension of the autonomous area proposed by the regime. There was a simple reason: The demographics had changed so much since 1970 that Kirkuk no longer had sufficient Kurdish population to be considered part of the Kurdish autonomous region. Barzani accused Saddam of "Arabizing Kurdistan" and of dragging his feet on completing the census. Fighting broke out again, and two Kurdish towns of about 20,000–25,000 inhabitants were destroyed. Napalm was allegedly used routinely.[49]

In 1974, during the ongoing joint investigation between the University of Rochester and the University of Baghdad of the Iraqi methylmercury poisoning, Saddam actively pursued a plan to build a chemical plant. Iraq officials said they needed a facility to manufacture large quantities of vaccines to help develop agricultural and animal production, though research by Con Coughlin suggests that Saddam's initial interest was in biological weapons. Saddam's group was referred to the Pfaudler company of Rochester, New York, which specialized in the manufacture of equipment for mixing toxic chemicals. In 1976, Pfaudler presented a detailed proposal for a pilot plant. The Iraqis said they wanted to manufacture four highly toxic organic compounds: amiton, demeton, paraoxon, and parathion.[50]

Certainly, the scientists, both American and Iraqi, investigating the mercury seed grain poisoning had more to contend with than the science at hand in this tragedy. Just how reliable any of the data coming out of Iraq were is in question. At the time of the poisoning, the 1973 *Science* paper mentioned that the data would be important to the fishing industry. The United States, WHO, Canada, and Japan all had an interest in knowing what level of exposure would lead to adverse effects, and it appears they have continued to use the data to make assessments as to whether people exposed to methylmercury are suffering from toxicity. To track that down, at least in the United States, we need to take a trip into the United States court system, to one of the greatest matches of industry versus industry regulators.

CHAPTER 12

Fishing with the
FDA for Evidence in Iraq

T HE IRAQI SEED GRAIN POISONING and the questionable Iraqi-
controlled results emanating from it would prove central to a case
I learned about that would have far-reaching implications on how much
mercury would be allowed in fish. The case was heard in 1977 in the
United States District Court for the Northern District of Florida, Marianna Division, with Judge Winston E. Arnow presiding.

The FDA had sued Anderson Seafoods, Inc., because the company's swordfish were testing at mercury levels higher than the FDA's
safe limit at the time of 0.5 mcg/g. The swordfish and tuna industry had
already lost millions to the first mercury scare in the United States and
Canada in the early 1970s, and the companies involved would have to
do something soon or suffer even more losses. Swordfish had been
removed from the market briefly in the early 1970s, and the industry
was struggling to make a comeback. An allowable mercury limit of 0.5
mcg/g (the FDA and EPA's benchmark for commercial and noncommercial fish) would make only about half of the swordfish catch fit for
sale, as the average mercury level in the fish at that time—and still
today—was 1 mcg/g.

Despite the poisonings of methylmercury that had occurred around
the world, clear standards still had not been set for this toxicant in the
1970s. This was the case for mercury in seed grain, fish, pollutants
released to the atmosphere, medications, cosmetics, and other food
items. In addition, as we've seen, there was heated controversy even
many years later over what symptoms and health effects constituted
toxicity in humans.

The World Health Organization, along with Thomas Clarkson's

University of Rochester team, went to Iraq to develop the standards. They needed to determine what level of exposure would begin to cause harm to humans and from that to extrapolate at what level the mercury found in fish would constitute a risk to the public. The Iraqis, on the other hand, had to find ways to ease the interrogations of the international community about the poisoning. After an editorial appeared in the June 1972 *British Medical Journal* criticizing the Iraqi poisoning and the manufacturers and distributors of dangerous chemicals, the Iraqis responded:

> Many of those who were graded as "severe," being completely paralyzed and bedridden, improved greatly and began to be independent in caring for themselves and walking around after several weeks of patient physical therapy. Partial sight was recovered by some and partial hearing by others. This happened not only in the children who received treatment with chelating agents or polythiol resin but also those who had no drug therapy. . . . We shall be publishing these findings soon, but whatever the reason for this improvement we are certain that the international organizations could give great help in the field of rehabilitation. WHO should immediately direct its efforts in that way rather than believing that nothing can be done for the large number of crippled patients.[1]

WHO, the Iraqi government, and Clarkson's Rochester group subsequently studied several populations affected by the poisoning and reported the results promptly, as we've seen, in the 1973 article in *Science*, which addressed mostly adults. One of the first papers on exposure of Iraqi mothers and their infants, unfortunately including only fifteen mother-infant pairs, was by Laman Amin-Zaki and Clarkson, based on blood specimens collected between March 6 and November 14, 1972. "The lowest concentration of mercury in an individual blood sample associated with maternal signs and symptoms of poisoning was 300 ppb [parts per billion; mcg/l]," they concluded. They also stated that all mothers who had measured blood levels in excess of 400 mcg/l exhibited signs and symptoms of poisoning. Clinical manifestations of methylmercury poisoning were seen in six of the fifteen mothers and at least six of the fifteen infants. In five severely affected infants there was gross impairment of motor and mental development. The rest of the infants, they concluded, would need to be followed through their lives to see if further developmental effects occurred. The most common symptoms of the mothers affected were malaise, a feeling of general body discomfort, vague muscle and joint pains, loss of sensation around the mouth and in the extremities, weakness, exaggerated reflexes, and visual changes. The paper also noted that some of the women with very affected infants seemed themselves to be without complaint of symptoms.[2]

It was not until 1978 that a *British Medical Journal* article led by Laman Amin-Zaki reported on a two-year follow-up of forty-nine pediatric patients who had been victims of the Iraqi poisoning. The subjects were divided into four crude categories by severity of symptoms—mild, moderate, severe, and very severe. The mercury level at which the symptoms first began to appear was not available, so it could only be estimated based on extrapolation from other evidence. Six children fell into the mild category, and their symptoms were mainly subjective— malaise, headache, insomnia, paresthesia, weakness, blurring of vision, gastrointestinal disturbances, and hyperreflexia (the jerking movements that occur when a doctor strikes you with a hammer on the knee, but exaggerated—an indicator of possible brain injury). The researchers also found no apparent relation between the severity of signs and symptoms and the mercury concentrations. This may seem odd, but because there are genetic differences among individuals and the mercury levels in relation to the dose and time of dose were not uniform, this would be expected. Then there is the Tikriti factor. Dr. Tikriti gave out only the information that he or his superiors agreed to give out. This could also account for erratic data. As for the miraculous recovery of the more severe patients, the report's authors stated, "The two-year follow-up study indicates that those who were initially disabled, paralyzed, and bedridden improved greatly with time and began to be independent in caring for themselves and walking around. We have no doubt that physiological function improves or even recovers completely."[3]

I asked Philippe Grandjean, the Harvard mercury researcher and author of the Faroes studies, two questions: (1) What is the probability that an infant born with a mercury level of greater than 250 mcg/l would be normal? (2) What is the probability that an infant who went blind as a result of mercury poisoning would see again? He answered, "The highest number we saw in the Faroes was 351 mcg/l. That child was within normal range on the neurodevelopmental tests given, but Minamata kids with that level of exposure would have severe problems—we're still trying to find reasons for the differences in vulnerability. Any sensory deficit that is due to developmental toxicity is unlikely to be reversible. You only get one chance to develop a brain."[4]

In other words, children who were blinded by mercury were blinded through possibly irreversible processes. Miraculous recoveries of paralyzed and blinded children were unlikely to occur. Most intriguing was the fact that there appeared to be a tremendous difference between individuals in their ability to tolerate methylmercury. This observation is consistent with what we see in methylmercury-exposed humans of various ages today.

What became confusing to me was that even though the Iraqi seed grain poisoning studies did not determine the lowest level of mercury that resulted in symptoms or signs of mercury, somehow the FDA and many health care people thought they did. It was the minimal-clinical-effect level (MCEL) and the no-observable-effect level (NOEL) that were important to identify in setting standards for mercury exposure. The MCEL was the level at which signs and symptoms began to occur in the most sensitive individual. The NOEL was the level of mercury below which no one was affected. The Iraqi studies, limited even if you take the data for face value, did not determine a NOEL or an MCEL. This is because they did not look at individual patients and instead lumped people into groups. More sensitive individuals could be in a group with the less sensitive, and therefore would not be identified by such a group-type study. Furthermore, there was no control population.

Even in 1974, the FDA still recommended that fish with mercury concentrations greater than 0.5 mcg/g (ppm) not be sold on the commercial market. This level was arbitrarily set during the Canadian mercury scare that spread into the United States in 1970. This left the canned tuna industry at a loss as to how to keep the levels down in cans that contained some of the larger and higher-mercury-contaminated species.

Because the FDA recognized that the amount of mercury in swordfish being sold commercially was higher than the limit the agency had set, it filed suit against Anderson Seafoods, Inc., a major swordfish proprietor, in 1977, for exceeding the FDA standard. Anderson countersued, and hearings began in mid-August of that year. This became the landmark case that ultimately decided how much methylmercury would be allowed in fish. It would result in the FDA losing its 0.5 mcg/g allowable-mercury policy, to be replaced by 1 mcg/g, a substantial difference in its consequences. This action level for allowable mercury in fish has been an impediment to change ever since.

The FDA contended that under the Enforcement Act swordfish distributed by Anderson were adulterated because they contained more than 0.5 mcg/g of mercury. Anderson declared, on the contrary, that fish containing more than 0.5 mcg/g of mercury were not adulterated, and even up to the level of 2 mcg/g would still not be considered adulterated under the law.[5]

How could fish that failed to meet the standard set by the FDA not be adulterated? Here is how the judge summarized that aspect of the Enforcement Act: "This act provides in relevant part that food is deemed adulterated: If it bears or contains any poisonous or deleterious substance which may render it injurious to health; but in case the substance is not an added substance such food shall not be considered adulterated under this clause if the quantity of such substance in such food does not ordinarily render it injurious to health."[6]

Judge Arnow's summary of 1978 noted that the experts testifying expressed widely divergent opinions and conclusions concerning the effects of methylmercury in swordfish. The FDA felt that the MCEL for methylmercury in blood was 200 mcg/l. This was based on a poisoning that occurred after the Minamata disaster, in Niigata, Japan, in 1966. Anderson said it relied on the "recent studies in Iraq." The company's experts stated that the MCEL was 400 mcg/l. The Iraq studies, they said, were confined to "field testing" and involved "group" rather than "individual" data, made use of more modern testing techniques, and tested a population subjected to a wider range of mercury doses than previous studies.

In other words, to decide how much mercury could be allowed in fish, then, the industry and FDA needed to know how much mercury could be tolerated in humans without harmful effect. The industry used the Iraq data for this purpose. Here is what the judge said about it: "Anderson's witnesses and the Iraq research upon which they rely have shown by a preponderance of the evidence that the MCEL for methylmercury is 400 mcg/l."[7]

In the end, the judge decided that there was no reasonable possibility of injury to anyone's health from the consumption of swordfish containing 1 mcg/g or less of mercury (based on a notion of "normal" consumption patterns), and thus such swordfish could not be deemed adulterated on the basis of its mercury content. The judgment was duly entered in favor of the plaintiff, Anderson Seafoods, Inc. In other words, instead of enforcing the 0.5 mcg/g limit, the judge raised it to 1 mcg/g.

How had the judge reached the conclusion of an MCEL of 400 mcg/l, when the studies in Iraq were not designed to determine an MCEL, I wondered when I read the case summary and conclusions. Certainly, Thomas Clarkson would know how the studies were designed, as he was the lead American researcher in Iraq and had already written a number of papers, including one with Amin-Zaki, showing that symptoms occurred at lower levels of exposure. I therefore hunted down the *FDA vs. Anderson* case and requested the docket sheets. Clarkson did give a deposition, and it was for the FDA, it turned out, but to my dismay his deposition was sealed by order of the court and was never entered into evidence.

Fortunately, the case had been retired to the National Archives, I discovered, and Clarkson's deposition was evidently no longer under seal. I therefore was able to read his deposition along with a transcript of the four days of testimony, which ran some 1,140 pages.

The FDA began its case with a marine geochemist who told the court that there were manmade and natural sources of mercury in the ocean. Unfortunately, government agencies had not tested mercury levels in ocean sediments more than three miles from shore. This posed a strategic problem for the FDA, as the fishing industry was arguing that swordfish were not near the human sources of mercury and therefore their methylmercury levels were "natural."

If the fishing industry was able to win acceptance from the court that a substance was "natural"—as it was able to in this case—it could essentially get around the statute. "Naturally occurring" status for methylmercury requires the industry to prove only that the amount that is found in the fish is not "ordinarily" injurious.

An array of FDA witnesses testified for the first two days of the trial on a variety of aspects of mercury, fish, and human health. One witness, for example, testified that though 90 percent of the swordfish taken off California were caught fifty miles off shore, they ate fish that reside within three miles of shore, where human-generated pollution existed (which led to the high concentration of mercury in these predators).

A key FDA witness who addressed the effects of methylmercury on humans was Frank Lu, MD, the scientific secretary for WHO. He was described as a "toxicologist" but did not have a PhD in toxicology. Anderson lawyers questioned this designation and would consider him only as a medical expert. In his testimony, Dr. Lu was able to address the absorption of methylmercury in humans and how it was distributed throughout the body. He gave his opinion, based on his review of the literature, as to the lowest blood level of methylmercury that had been associated with overt clinical symptoms of intoxication: 200 mcg/l—a figure, he said, he based on findings from the poisoning in Niigata, Japan, and from the WHO study of Iraq.

In the trial, the Niigata data was heavily critiqued because the MCEL was calculated by "extrapolation," using data from only two individuals. In other words, the scientists did not test the blood when the symptoms began but later used a calculation to estimate what the mercury levels probably had been when the symptoms began. Furthermore, the machine that was used to conduct the tests, it was decided, was inaccurate—by as much as 200 percent. Dr. Lu stated that WHO estimated an MCEL of 200 mcg/l based on the subjective symptom of paresthesia. Placing the standard safety factor of 10 into the equation, WHO determined the acceptable daily intake (ADI) for mercury to be 30 mcg/day.[8] Neither WHO nor the Rochester group had done the type of study that could accurately determine the MCEL, thus the estimation.

Thirty mcg per day of mercury would be the equivalent of half a 170g-can of albacore tuna a day if the can contained 0.35 mcg/g Hg (0.35 mcg/g × 85g=30 mcg).[9] The current EPA advice for a 132-pound (60-kilogram) person would be to consume less than 6 mcg/day of mercury. The average consumer of fish among my patients ate three times the current EPA daily dose guideline—some even ten times that level.

Dr. Lu declared something that I had not known was ever argued until reading the trial transcript. He recognized that there were nonovert symptoms of methylmercury poisoning and felt that they were a part of the methylmercury exposure profile. This is also what the Japanese and the Canadian Indians had long recognized. Evidence on nonovert or nonspecific symptoms, which my patients had, was what I was looking for—such symptoms do indeed exist. They are also easily denied by the industries responsible for polluting.

The cross-examination of Dr. Lu by Robert Lasky, Anderson's lawyer, was rigorous and punctuated by questions about hypothetical case scenarios. Lasky was able to get Dr. Lu to admit that there had never been a reported case of mercury poisoning from pelagic fish (fish that live in the open sea) in the United States. This determination was still echoed by industry and the FDA in 2008. The FDA Web site identified nonspecific symptoms associated with mercury toxicity but did not declare the human blood level at which they occur. If nonspecific symptoms were part of the mercury toxicity profile, as the FDA Web site indicates and the FDA's witness, Dr. Lu, testified, why are they not used today to determine whether someone is likely suffering from too much mercury exposure? If these symptoms were recognized, then I have many individuals who could be considered mercury poisoned by eating these large fish.

The Iraq data was more reliable than Niigata's, Dr. Lu testified, but the WHO report did not permit the analysis required to identify a minimal- or no-effect level from the Iraqi poisoning. WHO placed the study subjects into groups according to their estimated intake of mercury. Some of the more sensitive people were grouped with the less sensitive. The analysis was made according to the symptoms in a group and did not identify individual cases. This group-type study, therefore, would not reveal the entire spectrum of mercury effects for individuals. All one could conclude from such a study was where the level at which the group was not showing symptoms became statistically significant.

In order to show the court that there were people in the United States who ate enough fish for accumulating mercury levels to be of concern, the FDA called Michael Weitzman, regional manager of franchise operations of Weight Watchers International, to the stand. The organization had been strongly encouraging participants to eat five fish meals per week; for lunch the recommended portion size was three to four ounces, and for dinner the recommended portion size for women and children was four to six ounces and for men six to eight ounces.

The FDA lawyers failed to inquire whether this diet had led to elevated mercury levels or health complaints. But then, the term "ordinarily" was also in the statute. The Weight Watchers group was not considered ordinary, and the industry lawyers would go on to make sure that they were not deemed ordinary by the judge.

One of the last witnesses to take the stand for the FDA was Bernard Weiss, professor of radiation biology and biophysics at the University of Rochester. He testified that the Rochester team had worked in Iraq under "relatively adverse circumstances." He said, "The Iraq data had shown that the mothers whose hair level was between 100 and 400 mcg/g [this would correspond to approximately 400–1,600 mcg/l in blood] produced children with considerable overt neurological and behavioral deficits. Retarded language development was observed in 70 percent of these children, and this is without statistics, because Dr. Marsh and Dr. Myers [Rochester researchers] were looking for clear, overt, unquestionable signs of toxicity."

Dr. Weiss did not agree with WHO's acceptable daily intake standard of 30 mcg/day. He thought it should be much lower:

> That estimate was based on overt clinical damage, and we know that a lot of brain damage can take place before symptoms bloom into clinical detectability. Second, the ADI also does not take into account the possibility of long-term damage, damage that may occur to the fetus and not be expressed until perhaps late in life, as the Japanese experience seems to indicate or suggest. Thirdly, the clinical evidence is also deficient because even in Japan, which has the longest experience, the children have not been examined with the same thoroughness, say, that they would be examined at the university medical school diagnostic clinic.[10]

After two days of the trial, the FDA abruptly rested its case. It was now Anderson's turn.

CHAPTER 13

Fishing with the Industry for Evidence in Iraq

T HE ANDERSON TRIAL WOULD TURN OUT TO BE the trial that set FDA policy for the past three decades on how much methylmercury is allowed in fish on the commercial market.[1] But so far, the FDA's top witness, Thomas Clarkson, hadn't appeared, and the FDA had not built as strong a case for the dangers of methylmercury in fish as it could have.

On day three of *United States of America vs. Anderson Seafoods, Inc.*, absent the availability of Clarkson for the FDA, Anderson began to call its witnesses. Charles Anderson himself, owner of Anderson Seafoods, was the first to take the stand. He estimated that 90 to 95 percent of swordfish he took in would have a mercury content in excess of 0.5 mcg/g, the action level in place at the FDA at the time. He declared to the court that there was no economic way to maintain his swordfish business at that action level.

But the real counterattack began when Marvin Friedman of Allied Chemical Corporation took the stand for Anderson. He held a master's degree in food science from the Massachusetts Institute of Technology and a PhD in nutrition. He had just taken a position at Allied, but for the six years previous, he had been on the pharmacology faculty at the Medical College of Virginia. He had been conducting a little-known rat experiment using methylmercury, and he started his testimony by saying that there was no evidence that mercury intakes between 30 and 300 mcg/day caused any effects at all [in humans]. The Iraq study was very well done, Friedman claimed, and employed "quantitative sophisticated analytical instrumentation"; it could be used to establish a basis for regulatory decisions, he felt.

In his experiment, Friedman said, he fed rats either milk protein with methylmercury added or swordfish protein that already contained methylmercury.[2] The rats fed the swordfish gained more weight, while the milk-fed rats crossed their hind legs, which was a previously recognized sign of mercury toxicity in cats. Friedman's interpretation was that swordfish protein "contains factors which ameliorate the toxicity of methylmercury," and he hypothesized that selenium, which he said was found in swordfish, was this protective substance. Based on the results of his experiment, his belief that swordfish contained protective factors, and his interpretation of the Iraqi WHO data, he gave his opinion that the blood level of mercury below which humans would be unaffected was 500 mcg/l. One could consume 150 mcg of mercury per day without effects, he testified. He said one could actually consume 750 mcg/day, but a safety factor of five should be used, thus the figure of 150 mcg. He later admitted to the presiding judge, Winston Arnow (this was not a jury trial), that the acceptable daily intake of 150 mcg that he had come up with was a "judgment thing" on his part. Paresthesia was the most sensitive parameter of mercury toxicity, he claimed, but he later admitted he did not actually know much about the signs and symptoms of mercury toxicity.

Friedman said a dose-response curve (a range of doses corresponding to adverse effects) for mercury created by the Iraqi researchers was "very well done," and he voiced the opinion that the Iraqi data provided a no-effect level. FDA's counsel Eric Blumberg countered by asking Friedman to point out in the WHO report where it said a no-effect level had been established. Friedman was unable to do so.

Claiming that a blood mercury level had been established under which humans were not affected would not only be an error, it would, if accepted by the court, establish for industry a barrier against all future suits brought by people who claimed they suffered adverse effects below that level. The statement, if accepted as true, would also likely have an impact on cases of methylmercury poisonings that were still being argued in the courts and political venues in Canada, Japan, and elsewhere.[3]

The rigorous cross-examination continued, with Blumberg questioning Dr. Friedman's numbers, calculations, and opinions, while Friedman countered with conclusions obtained from mercury studies carried out in other countries until Judge Arnow finally stopped the questioning to ask Friedman, "What are you talking about on blood levels?" FDA counsel Blumberg answered, "I'm not sure where he was talking, Your Honor. I was in Iraq. He's carried me all over the world."[4]

Friedman also had to admit to the court that his selenium–protective effect theory of swordfish was, in his words, "not supported by experimental data at all." Under cross-examination, he did not appear to know if swordfish in general contained selenium.[5] He could not account for the chemistry of his theory and had not tested the selenium content in the fish. He also did not know the caloric intake of the milk-fed versus the swordfish-fed rats, he admitted, as he never quantified their food intake,[6] yet he drew a favorable conclusion for the swordfish industry, anyway.

I should mention that in such court trials, those accepted as expert witnesses can offer any opinion they believe is true. They cannot be accused of lying necessarily, or of committing perjury. One can only say that they are not credible, or that they have been unethical. At this point in the trial, it was left to the FDA lawyers to counter any arbitrary statements from the industry experts. The FDA experts that could counter with knowledge of their own were in short supply, unfortunately.

After Friedman came Vincent Guinn. He had been a consultant to the World Health Organization and the International Atomic Energy Agency of the United Nations. He was retained by the defense as an expert in analytical chemistry. He tested museum samples of oceangoing tuna and swordfish and compared them to fresh fish. The mercury found in the fresh tuna and swordfish were of natural origin, he claimed, because the mercury levels of the museum samples were comparable, which indicated that mercury was not from human sources of pollution. On cross-examination, it was learned that he had only tested one museum sample of a swordfish head and seven museum samples of tuna. The "fresh" tuna was from a can, and he had no way of knowing where the fish originated—he "just went to the supermarket and picked them up."[7] The exchange over this issue was important. The industry lawyers were trying to establish an opinion that methylmercury in swordfish was natural. If they succeeded, they would only have to prove that "ordinary" consumption was not injurious to health.

Anderson's counsel continued with a parade of selected experts by calling John Crispin-Smith to the stand. He was an associate professor of pharmacology, toxicology, radiation biology, and biophysics at the Rochester School of Medicine and Dentistry. He had been involved in the research of the methylmercury poisoning in Iraq, as well as studies of populations in Peru and American Samoa that had high intakes of marine fish. He also said he had visited Japan, to "study further the results of the investigations of the Japanese investigators."[8]

Crispin-Smith thought the Iraqi data was "superb" because new analytical methods for testing were more accurate than they had been in the past. He did not feel the Japanese data were accurate, and thought his Iraqi analytical methods and data were a "better basis for reaching conclusions."[9] He went on to assert that the FDA had relied on the Japanese data to set its original 0.5 mcg/g action level for methylmercury content in fish. He now wanted the Iraqi data to be used as the basis for a revised action level, as it would allow less stringent standards for methylmercury in fish and higher consumption of methylmercury.

Because of more accurate methodologies and machinery, Crispin-Smith also claimed that the Iraqi data would allow use of a lower safety factor in determining acceptable limits of exposure. Instead of ten, five could be used. The safety factor, you recall, is a number that accounts for variability and unforeseen factors. It serves as a buffer to the actual toxic level of exposure identified in the study.

Crispin-Smith had been in Iraq twice, he testified, for one month each time, to oversee lab testing in Baghdad. He did not examine patients, nor did he say that he even spoke to any of them.[10] He was in charge of the lab tests, but he did not have a chain of possession for the specimens—it was Dr. Tikriti who was providing all the data.[11] Crispin-Smith went on to testify that there was no patient with any sign or symptom related to methylmercury intake who had a blood mercury level lower than 500 mcg/l. He told the court how he extrapolated the data to predict the level at which symptoms would occur. By his math, the lowest observable effect level was 1,000 mcg/l.

Whew! Dr. Crispin-Smith was bold, for sure. But his conclusion was shaky. The Iraqis did not fill out questionnaires for the patients, and the people were looked at in groups and not as individuals. You can't identify the lowest observable effect level using groups, because the said effect and its corresponding mercury level, is averaged out over the varying individuals among the group.[12]

Crispin-Smith went on to give the opinion that the Iraqi data were able to identify a minimal-clinical-effect level at which symptoms might first begin to appear, and that was a blood level of 400 mcg/l for infants and 500 mcg/l for everyone else, which would correspond to an allowable weekly intake (AWI) of 840 mcg.[13] A weekly intake of 840 mcg under today's standards would allow a 132-pound (60-kilogram) person to consume fourteen (6-ounce, or 170-gram) cans of albacore tuna per week. This may sound like an incredible amount to those who do not like fish, but I have seen people who claim to consume more than that. They were not feeling very well, however. I am sure the industry knew those folks existed, too; it would, therefore, have to claim that those high-end consumers were not "ordinary."

To do that, Dr. Crispin-Smith calculated what he deemed to be a "worst-case scenario" for the court. He felt that four servings of six ounces of swordfish and four servings of six ounces of tuna per week was the worst case. Using the mercury levels available for these fish, he calculated that intake of fish to include 948 mcg of mercury per week.

This would be 113 percent of the allowable weekly intake of 840 mcg. But, because the methylmercury in swordfish accounted for only 90 percent of the total mercury, he claimed, and methylmercury is the "toxic" form of mercury to be concerned with, 90 percent of 948 was about 840, 100 percent of the average weekly intake he had claimed was safe. Even he commented that 100 percent was "unfortunate, as you don't like the numbers to come out quite as close as that."[14]

Separating methylmercury from the other mercury compounds in swordfish and tuna was not what the argument was really about, though, despite what he testified. The other mercury compounds had not been proven to be any safer than methylmercury at that time—or subsequently. But it was a good try, and the assumption allowed him to get his numbers absolutely perfect.

He went on to claim that the probability that a person existed in the United States with this consumption pattern would be one in forty million. He predicted that the blood level achieved by such a person would be 90 mcg/l, and that would be "only one-fourth of the minimal clinical effect level of 400 mcg/l." With this, Crispin-Smith concluded that there was no necessity for a guideline or action level with regard to mercury in pelagic oceangoing fish because there was no chance of there being any problems.[15]

The judge was concerned that Crispin-Smith did not allow for the higher mercury levels that could be found in swordfish, as some fish had mercury levels of more than 2 mcg/g. Judge Arnow was sharp to realize that Crispin-Smith's calculations were based on the mean level of mercury found in swordfish, and that Crispin-Smith's no-guideline-necessary conclusion was not protective for all.[16] The judge then asked Crispin-Smith to make a series of recalculations on the average mercury content in the fish until Crispin-Smith declared, "An expert witness is a man with an electronic calculator and a return ticket to New York."[17]

Blumberg on cross hammered Crispin-Smith with questions about where it was stated in the Iraqi studies that the zero effect level was 500 mcg/l. At one point Blumberg stated, "I don't believe you answered. Is it stated *in haec verba*, do you know what I'm saying, in precise words, that zero point five [500 mcg/l] is a no-effect level, or is that interpretation that you placed on the data?" Crispin-Smith answered with, "I would say it is an interpretation I placed on the data."[18]

When asked whether he had made contrary statements in his testimony compared to the 1973 *Science* article he had coauthored, Crispin-Smith explained that his views since then had changed—his testimony expressed his present view that the Iraqi data did not agree with the Japanese findings of a minimum-effect level of 200 mcg/l. Blumberg then asked Crispin-Smith if Thomas Clarkson had changed his view in that direction as well.

Lasky objected: "If Clarkson is going to be here as a witness, he can testify."

Judge Arnow: "If he's going to be here, the objection is sustained."

Great! The industry experts continued to give their "opinions" and the FDA lawyers gave no adequate counter-arguments. Where was Clarkson? He should know what was done in those studies and how they were conducted. He was a consultant for the industry as well as the FDA.

Although Crispin-Smith may have changed his mind about how to interpret the data, the methods for the studies remained the same, and, therefore, a no-effect level or minimal-effect level would still not have been possible to establish. Without a control population, and proper evaluations for each study subject, the significance of the nonspecific symptoms or the full spectrum of effects could not be determined.

One of the next experts to take the stand was Solomon Margolin, a PhD in physiology, biochemistry, and genetics and president and chairman of the board at AMR Biological Research, Inc., a contract research organization that conducted biological research, both basic and clinical, on behalf of the pharmaceutical, chemical, and cosmetic industries. He was retained as an expert in pharmacology and toxicology by the defense. When asked to give his expert opinion as to what he "believed" to be an allowable daily intake for mercury, he stated, "Without introducing any so-called safety factors, which are arbitrary numbers, the direct value is 800 mcg/day." A safety factor "was a matter of judgement in terms of overall policy," he argued. "Based on pure science, a safety factor was not necessary. A safety factor is only used in terms of practical development of public health policy." His conclusion was that the "practical level" of mercury allowable in fish should be 2 mcg/g as a matter of public health policy.[19]

I myself felt tunnel vision coming on with mention of that dose. Yes, that was no mistake—he said it a few times: 800 mcg/day. Ninety-three cans of albacore tuna per week! That just about covers any eventuality for the tuna industry. That would break the all-time canned tuna consumption record. Don't anyone try this at home. Seriously, a steady diet like that would result in a 132-pound (60-kilogram) person having a mercury level of about 600 mcg/l. There is no legitimate scientific literature today that would support a continued blood mercury level of 600 mcg/l as being without harm.

The next researcher to testify for Anderson was Dr. David O. Marsh, a neurologist from the University of Rochester. He was involved in the assessment of the neurological and toxicological consequences of the methylmercury poisoning in Iraq and examined subjects in studies in Samoa and Peru. Like others before him, he expressed an opinion that there was a no-effect level for adults, which was 500 mcg/l and was derived from the Iraqi data. He also claimed that only a safety factor of five was needed, because "many of the uncertainties that existed have decreased." He also agreed with Crispin-Smith that a guideline for allowable mercury in fish should be 2 mcg/g. "There's never been a single case of methylmercury poisoning caused by ocean fish and diagnosed in this country or in any other country," he claimed.[20]

As for the study on the children, when asked whether the data allowed for the establishment of a no-effect level, Marsh replied, "The study concluded that there was an effect level." His view of minimum abnormality was certainly a disturbing one: "Children who we determined were mildly affected were children looking normal, running around, behaving normally. And only with the most minimal retardation. They were a little slower to walk, perhaps a little slower to talk. They had increased frequency of seizures compared with the control group. Their height was slightly shorter. Their head circumference was slightly smaller. These were all very, very minimal effects."[21]

Of course mental retardation, small head circumference, seizures, and slow to walk and talk are certainly not minimal effects by normal medical standards, or by anyone else's; they are serious in themselves and likely indicate a lot of damage to those infants before those effects were seen.

On cross-examination, Marsh's methods of assessment came under scrutiny. His tests for peripheral vision employed a ball and plastic cup as instruments—a technique that does not allow for refined measurements. For his studies of mercury effects in Samoa and Peru, he admitted that he "did not do full psychological testing" or "detailed psychometric testing." As for how he did assess the people for the effects of mercury, he stated, "When one is faced with patients who speak another language, their ability to cooperate and carry out testing is a very useful rough way of knowing whether they are mentally impaired or not."[22] Perhaps obedience to the test administrators, it seems, was his measure of intelligence.

So that was it for the industry's expert testimony. And the FDA's as well. Oh yes, Thomas Clarkson. Multiple changes were made to the dates when his testimony would take place. It seemed a kind of cat-and-mouse game, but it was unclear who was to blame, the industry or Clarkson himself. In the end, he could not make it to the trial because of other engagements and was only able to give a deposition out of court. The date for that, too, had to be rescheduled, at the request of Anderson's attorneys.[23]

The government argued with the court that if Clarkson's deposition were not admitted into evidence, the government's case would be "substantially prejudiced." So, to "preserve the record and avoid further delay," the government took a deposition on September 17 under protest by Anderson counsel, who then argued against allowing Clarkson's deposition into evidence. They said that the content of his deposition was irrelevant and that the FDA had not followed proper procedure for procuring a witness. A deposition did not allow examination or scrutinizing by the court, they pointed out, and they claimed it was inappropriate to have a discovery type of deposition post trial. Because Clarkson had been in the country for prolonged periods prior to the trial, he was therefore amenable to process. (He was available; therefore, the FDA was at fault for not getting him to trial.) After review of the laws and technical aspects thereof, and after hearing both sides, on October 31, 1977, Judge Arnow ordered that the deposition, having been taken for record purposes, be filed in the records but "sealed by the clerk of this court to be opened only pursuant to order of a competent court. Such deposition will not be used or considered as evidence in this case."[24]

Obviously, the industry lawyers were afraid of what he would say. After all, he was in charge of their methylmercury studies. When I saw in the docket sheets a list of all the objection letters being written, I asked for everything I thought significant, and the deposition was included. Here, then, is a summary of what the Anderson attorneys did not want heard.[25]

It started off with Anderson attorney Robert Lasky objecting to Clarkson being characterized as an expert in the field of toxicology with special expertise in the areas of mercury, methylmercury toxicity in humans, and the determination of mercury blood levels in humans. This objection seemed surprising to me, considering that Clarkson was the fishing industry's lead researcher for methylmercury in fish, had developed a mercury chelator for Dow, and had developed the methods used for testing blood and tissues that seemed to be so critical for getting the Iraqi data accepted in lieu of the Japanese data. Clarkson had been studying methylmercury since the 1960s and had traveled to just about every place in the world where there was a major mercury problem. It appears this was a warning to him.

Clarkson stated that he had been to Iraq six times. He was the principal investigator and in charge of the grants that paid for the studies. He was also responsible "from the University of Rochester's point of view for the scientific direction of the studies." He said that he asked John Crispin-Smith to help primarily for his expertise in identifying methylmercury, but Crispin-Smith and Marsh were never the principal investigators. Federal grants to cover expenses for his studies in Iraq were about $500,000 annually.

Clarkson was careful about what terminology he consented to. He agreed that "the lowest blood level which has been associated with 'overt clinical symptoms' and signs of methylmercury intoxication was

200 mcg/l." He based his opinion, he said, on the information from the Niigata outbreak, and that those results were consistent with the results from Iraq.

Clarkson confirmed that three main studies took place in Iraq. The first study was carried out by the University of Rochester in collaboration with the University of Baghdad in the early "outbreak" of the poisoning—when people began presenting with symptoms. This study did not identify cases of methylmercury poisoning, as the researchers did not ask the physician to diagnose it. In Clarkson's words, "What we asked them [the physicians] was to report paresthesia, ataxia, and so on. We then grouped the population according to their average methylmercury levels from very low to very high, and compared the reported signs and symptoms in each group with the methylmercury levels, what we call a frequency study. . . . Now this does not identify a person who is the most sensitive in that population." Clarkson was thus acknowledging, without directly doing so, that in this study it wasn't possible to determine a minimum-effect level.

The second study was carried out by WHO and involved almost two thousand subjects. Clarkson said that neither he nor anyone else from the University of Rochester, was involved. He explained that in the WHO study, "they did the same kind of thing, that is, a frequency study," and, he said, the WHO results agreed with the results of his Rochester study. WHO additionally classified the subjects into "extreme, moderate, and so on" and found subjective evidence of methylmercury poisoning in more than twenty females who had maximum hair levels below 100 mcg/g (about 400mcg/l in blood). The WHO researchers thought that one should diagnose what they called a subjective methylmercury poisoning—a syndrome mild in form that was related to subjective complaints by the patients. He later described these "health complaints" as nonspecific in nature, and although he could not remember all of them, he identified some as being paresthesia, headache, joint pains, and malaise.

This was what I was looking for. The lesser symptoms being seen at levels below this 400 mcg/l barrier. If overt symptoms were seen at 200 mcg/l, then the lesser symptoms were most likely seen below 200 mcg/l. This also confirmed what Dr. Tikriti had said. Had Dr. Clarkson stated this at the trial itself, the allowable level of mercury in fish might well have been kept at 0.5 mcg/g, and the swordfish industry would not have continued to exist for long. This would have posed a challenge to the other industries that sold large predatory fish, including the canned tuna industry that used the larger and higher-mercury-content tuna such as albacore and ahi.

The third study was of the infant-mother pairs. Clarkson stated, "We did not identify cases of methylmercury poisoning in the infant, as the signs and symptoms could be due to other causes, and the proof that they are caused by methylmercury depends upon the appropriate choice of a control group, and the comparison of the size of these abnormalities in the exposed and controlled group." In other words, they could not establish the full spectrum of mercury toxicity or the no-effect level since they had no control group.

A curious finding of the analysis of hair levels as stated in the *Science* article is that "the average duration of exposure, according to the patients' report, was 48 days and that computed from analysis of hair samples for the same patients was 66 days."[26] Clarkson could not say why this discrepancy was present though he did agree that the results suggested the consumption period was longer than what patients had stated.

This introduces the idea that Dr. Tikriti, the researchers, or the patients may have erred or have not given full disclosure on the particulars of the poisoning, such as how long the patients were exposed, how much bread was eaten, and so forth. Scientists continued to have trouble making statistical sense of the Iraqi data, which was not always consistent. This makes even more dubious the idea that one could abstract from this event a minimum-effect level.

Clarkson, it seemed clear, essentially did not agree with Crispin-Smith's and Marsh's assessment of the Iraqi data. He stated numerous times that the Iraqi studies were not designed to define the minimal-clinical-effect level or a no-effect level. He was allowed to reiterate on cross-examination by the FDA counsel that symptoms were reported in blood levels below 400 mcg/l. He also did not agree with the claims that fish had some sort of protective property against methylmercury poisoning.

Clarkson mentioned twice a report or survey that a man named McDuffy presented at Rochester, a survey of people on the Weight Watchers diet who consumed fish according to the recommendations given in the Weight Watchers pamphlets. He disclosed that some of the people in the survey apparently had mercury levels between 50 mcg/l and 100 mcg/l by consuming swordfish and tuna. So here was evidence of a group of high-end fish consumers. Perhaps they were not "ordinary," but they did indeed exist. This is the type of consumer I discovered among my patient population.

During the trial, Leonard Goldwater—the author of the book *A History of Quicksilver*—gave testimony. He was asked by the Anderson attorney if he knew of a case of mercury poisoning from consuming ocean fish, as disclosed in his deposition. I should reiterate that the industry had said, and continues to say today, that there has never been a case of mercury poisoning by consuming ocean fish in the United States. Of course, we now know this is the mercury toxicity diagnosis that excludes the lesser symptoms. In other words, the public does not have mercury toxicity unless the industry says they have mercury toxicity. Goldwater, though, said he knew of one case, that of a woman who ate swordfish, who used the pseudonym Bettye Russow (or as it was misspelled Rousseau). Goldwater was asked if he had examined her, and he said no. Industry attorneys then asked that all the testimony about that individual be stricken from the record. The case, though, had been reported in the literature; therefore, the judge overruled this motion.[27] But nothing further was said about her at the trial. Her not wanting to be identified and the misspelling of her pseudonym made her lost to follow-up, allowing industry to claim that no one in the United States ate enough swordfish for its mercury level to be of concern. According to a 1972 article about Russow in *Nutrition Today*, her doctor thought she had a textbook case of methylmercury poisoning. She had been on a weight-reducing diet, which called for her to consume 4 ounces of swordfish for lunch and 10 ounces at dinner. She was eating about 12.5 ounces total. She weighed 165 pounds (75 kilograms), and was thirty-eight years old. After losing 45 pounds, she continued this diet off and on for about five years while maintaining a weight of 120–125 pounds. During this time, she began experiencing lethargy, headaches, blurred vision, tremor in her hands, a marked decline in her memory, dizziness, unsteady gait, impaired speech and writing, and difficulty with word finding. Her hair level after being off swordfish for five months was 42 mcg/g. (This would correspond to about 168 mcg/l in her blood.) Her estimated mercury intake with this diet would have been about 340 mcg/day. Certainly higher than WHO's 30-mcg/d acceptable level in the 1970s or today's EPA acceptable dose of less than 5.5 mcg/day. After stopping swordfish consumption, her symptoms resolved, according to the article.[28]

Despite this, the FDA failed to inquire about the health effects of this type of diet and level of mercury exposure, and failed to adequately use the Weight Watchers' mercury levels or any part of the Weight Watchers' exposed population at the trial to stress that there were people with significant exposure to methylmercury from consuming fish in the United States. When Clarkson was asked about the symptoms that occur at these lower levels of exposure and whether the people recovered, he answered, "some of these people have recovered, but it's not a hundred percent."[29]

Clarkson made an interesting statement in his deposition on the Iraqi data and the survey of Weight Watchers: "These two situations bother me, and perhaps I'm going beyond your question, but in this sense, there would appear to be a risk. I cannot establish the magnitude of the risk, and this is what concerns me about the release of swordfish on the market again."[30]

This was indeed a strong statement. To this day, I have never seen anywhere in print that, for whatever reason, he said anything like this again.

With the Clarkson testimony disallowed, the judge ruled in favor of Anderson Seafoods Inc., and the FDA and WHO have been relying on "data" from the Iraq incident and the results of this trial to tell us how much methylmercury is allowed in our fish ever since. The MCEL, according to the lead researcher in the Iraq investigation, was not established because the studies were not designed to do that. Symptoms did occur at levels less than 200 mcg/l. Regardless, the Anderson "experts" were able to convince the judge that a minimal- or no-effect level had been established—a high one at that.

The studies in Iraq were based on handpicked "data" by Dr. Tikriti of the Iraqi Ministry of Health. It was a poisoning that was suspicious at best. No formal epidemiologic study was completed. The "minor" symptoms would simply be ignored. The "minimal" signs were not so minimal. The Iraqis had reason to downplay this incident to keep WHO and the international community from further investigation. Dow and the fishing industry had a stake in the outcome, as well.

After the trial, in 1980, researchers led by Marsh, Myers, and Clarkson, along with Amin-Zaki and Tikriti, published another paper together. It discussed the clinical and toxicological data on twenty-nine infants in the Iraq poisoning. They stated that standardized questionnaires were used but did not go into detail as to what was on them. They concluded that the small number of infant-mother pairs in their study did not allow them to identify a specific "threshold" maternal hair concentration below which there would be no adverse effects in either mother or infant. They did see effects, they said, at the lower levels but could not obtain a dose curve for them.[31]

Interestingly, later papers to come out of Iraq began to take a different turn, and symptoms and effects at lower levels began to be reported. In 1980, a paper appeared in the *Postgraduate Medical Journal*, written by Bakir, Tikriti, Damluji, and a nuclear scientist who is an important and historic figure in Iraq, Hussein al-Shahristani. They concluded that the Dow resin Clarkson used did not change the clinical outcomes of the patients and that there was a "mild group" category whose subjective symptoms consisted of irritability, malaise, headache, generalized aches and pains, muscle weakness, abdominal discomfort, metallic taste in the mouth, sore gums, memory loss, anxiety, and paresthesias. The mild-category people had lower mercury levels, but the dose-symptom relationship was inconstant. The researchers did not say at what level these symptoms occurred. The mild to moderate cases and a few of the severe cases improved, but the researchers concluded that the severe and very severe cases did not improve.[32]

By 1987, David Marsh, with Clarkson, Amin-Zaki and Tikriti, concluded, based on more extensive testing and questions asked through Iraqi interpreters that a much lower hair mercury level than previously acknowledged was associated with adverse effects in children—6 mcg/g. (This would correspond to a blood level of about 24 mcg/l.) They concluded, "If confirmed by further studies, the implications for high fish consumers are serious. A hair level of only 6 mcg/g can be attained by long-term daily consumption of a 3-ounce meal of tuna (assumed to contain 0.3 mcg/g of mercury as methyl mercury)."[33]

At this point, the Iraqi literature began to lose its usefulness to the fishing industry.* But, because the earlier Iraqi reports suggested that one could have much higher exposure to mercury without effects, and those were the reports used and misinterpreted by industry experts in the court trial that decided how much mercury should be in fish, the

---

*So what happened to the scientists after the Iraqi poisoning?

With the fall of Saddam, Dr. Tikriti moved from Iraq to the United States in 2003. Farhan Bakir, Saddam's personal physician, was "forced into early retirement." He told reporters for *Nature* that he feared for his safety, and he left Iraq in 1981. Although he was said to be in California, according to the California Medical Board, he did not answer my e-mails when asked about this historic event. By 2006, the post office gave a forwarding address in Saudi Arabia.[34]

Damluji and Amin-Zaki, who were husband and wife, moved away from Iraq some time after the poisoning incident and are deceased, according to Dr. Tikriti.

Dr. Al-Shahristani, a nuclear chemist, in the autumn of 1979 became one of two chief scientific advisers to Iraq's nuclear program. He spoke out publicly against Saddam's nuclear program and "serious violations of human rights." He was arrested; tortured for three weeks, including being hung upside down for hours; then placed in solitary confinement for ten years. He escaped in 1991 during the Gulf War and is now heading Iraq's Scientific Academy. He recently stated, "The Academy will also revive Iraqi talents for the good of humanity after decades of abuse of Iraqi scientists under Saddam Hussein's regime." He also has not answered my e-mail inquiries.[35]

mercury action level of 1 mcg/g for commercial fish in the United States has remained unchallenged.

With the judge's decision in 1977, the mercury content of swordfish and tuna became for years an issue of the past, and the "mercury scare of 1970" simply sank to the depths of ancient history. The Bettye Russows never went away, though. They just weren't recognized.

CHAPTER 14

From American Samoa to Peru

THE MERCURY SCARE THAT BEGAN IN 1970 in Canada and spread to the United States was a difficult time for the fishermen who sold mercury-laden fish. An FDA mercury action level of 0.5 mcg/g imposed on their catch was almost impossible to comply with for those selling some types of tuna, swordfish, and other fish with the highest mercury content, and difficult for many others. Losses to the tuna and swordfish industry were felt immediately and ran in the millions of dollars. The fishing industry needed to fight back with its own investigation, to prove to the public that its products were safe to eat in quantity. American Samoa and Peru turned out to be good locations for this task.[1] It was Thomas Clarkson who initiated these studies and directed their progress. In the 1977 Anderson trial, these studies were referred to repeatedly by industry, purportedly to show there were no effects from mercury at the level of exposure that can be encountered by routinely consuming commercial fish.

In looking closely at the studies conducted and the testimonies given, I began to realize that these researchers were not likely to find effects of methylmercury in any fish-consuming population. First, they did not know the full spectrum of symptoms from their Iraqi studies, and, second, they did not investigate "subjective" effects of methylmercury poisoning. As revealed by David Marsh at the trial, the researchers in the Samoa and Peru studies "did not do full psychological testing" or "detailed psychometric testing." Marsh simply claimed, as we saw, that the study subjects' "ability to cooperate and carry out testing is a very useful rough way of knowing whether they are mentally impaired or not."[2] One might wonder, if he did only limited testing, did he do much in the way of observing? Regardless, these studies were almost impossible to find in the literature. Thanks to Katy Mahaffey and her EPA librarians, we can now take a look at what they were all about. It appears that the research team was trying to eliminate the notion that subjective symptoms such as fatigue, headache, muscle pain, and the like occur before overt symptoms ensue. It was a convenient practice that the fisheries industries and others with a vested interest in minimizing mercury's effects could embrace: they would not want the toxicity profile expanded to include the lesser symptoms, as doing that could incur further regulation on their industry in order to protect public health.

The grants used for the study of Samoan-based fishery workers, which commenced in 1972, came from a number of federal and science agencies, as well as a lobbying group for the fishing industry, the Tuna Research Foundation.[3]

American Samoa, a location halfway around the world, might seem a strange place to commission the study that was begun here in 1972, but there's more of a connection than might meet the eye. When Captain T. F. Darden, U.S. Navy, wrote a report about American Samoa in 1951, on the occasion of administration of the island passing from the Department of the Navy to the Department of the Interior, it had a population of 5,700 people. The United States had gained possession of the island in 1900 and maintained a strategic naval base there, but aside from that, Captain Darden commented, "It is difficult to conceive of any nation gaining economic or financial benefit from American Samoa." At that time, its only export aside from handicrafts was copra.[4]

Darden included in his report, however, that in 1948, U.S. Naval property was leased to Island Packers, Inc., for the purpose of conducting a fish cannery using Samoan labor. The company had been forced to cease operations because of a shortage of fish for processing, he said, and it had been sold to Wilbur-Ellis Company. It did not take long, though, for the companies that owned StarKist and Chicken of the Sea to see the opportunity and move in. An import food broker, Emmet J. Purcell, who worked many years for the Wilbur-Ellis Company and founded Purcell International in the 1950s, also had a long relationship with the French Sardine Company, the company that was later known as StarKist. He was likely a key figure in bringing these companies together in American Samoa. Also, in 1954, the Van Camp Company and the Tokyo Marine Products Corporation in American Samoa began a joint venture in fish processing there. The Van Camp Seafood Company, as their venture was later called, developed the Chicken of the Sea label. In 1963, the Van Camp Seafood Company was purchased by Ralston Purina, who then sold it to Tri-Union Seafoods, LLC, in 1997.[5]

The first Samoan group studied by the Rochester researchers consisted of eighty-eight men working on tuna fishing boats. The second group was made up of forty-five Samoans working in a tuna-packing factory. Blood methylmercury levels for the tuna fishermen were on average 64 mcg/l with a range of 5–265 mcg/l, and for the packers, an average of 35 mcg/l with a range of 8–147 mcg/l. The researchers reported that these adults reported no symptoms compatible with poisoning and showed no associated neurological abnormalities on examination. (As a reminder, the average mercury level in my study subjects was 14 mcg/l, with a high of 89 mcg/l.)[6]

A formal questionnaire for the patients was not reported, nor was it said whether one was used to ask the study subjects about symptoms. The questions that it was clear the researchers did ask were those associated with the more severe, overt forms of mercury toxicity such as vision changes, paresthesia, and deafness. Extensive neuropsychiatric testing was not performed, and no control group for comparison to the study subjects was mentioned.

Although American Samoa had a rough start to its cannery, since 1975, Chicken of the Sea and StarKist have exported billions of dollars' worth of canned tuna from there to the United States. The corporations operating in American Samoa went on to develop the largest and most productive tuna canneries in the world. The reported results of the Samoans' methylmercury and health surveys were certainly not going to be an impediment to investors in the canned tuna industry.[7]

According to a number of recent reports, an estimated 80 percent of tuna landed in the western Pacific area were caught by purse seine fishing vessels based in American Samoa. The offices of the vessel owners were based in California, and the owners themselves were longtime fishing families that had passed their business through generations of their relatives. Most tuna caught by the U.S. purse seine fleet in the region was processed in American Samoa by StarKist and Chicken of the Sea and subsequently sold in the United States. These American Samoa canneries currently supply about 50 percent of the U.S. market for canned tuna.[8]

The economy of American Samoa in 2003 was more than 85 percent dependent either directly or indirectly on the U.S. tuna and fishing processing industries, according to American Samoan congressman Eni Faleomavaega, and the two main canneries employ more than 74 percent of the island's workforce. Congressman Faleomavaega has made it clear how central he believes the U.S. tuna fishing industry is to his island's interests: "I have always believed that workers in American Samoa are the backbone of the U.S. tuna industry and I believe our canneries have an obligation to protect the future of our workers. I also believe the U.S. government has an obligation to protect our interests."[9]

Bias is a potential issue with any scientific study. Conducting an objective and reliable study of industry employees designed to determine whether the product those workers are producing or selling is safe, because the employees themselves are exposed to the product (in this case eating it), is always an adventure. The employees not only have a financial interest in the outcome of the study, but also may fear for their jobs or disapproval from their fellow workers if they declare any complaint of adverse health effects. In 1972, the action of the U.S. Food and Drug Administration would have been fresh in the minds of the canners and tuna fishermen of Samoa, as the mercury scare of 1970 led to the FDA testing of canned tuna. At the time, 12.5 million cans of tuna were withdrawn, and Americans were advised not to eat swordfish at all. "When the first scare headlines hit, sales in some areas dropped nearly 40 percent," reported Charles R. Carry, executive director of the Tuna Research Foundation in 1972. "We've made substantial recoveries but there are probably some people who will never go back to the product." Carry also advised the "skippers to avoid catching the larger tuna; they seem to run to higher levels of mercury. We've also suggested that they shun certain areas."[10]

The results of the Samoan study were presented at a conference in Spain in 1974, under the auspices of the Fábrica National de Moneda y Timbre (the Spanish royal mint). Spain was also concerned about the mercury and tuna issue; by 2004, Spain would become the third-largest producer of canned tuna in the world, and in the years 1978–1997 it was fourth among the top ten leading countries producing tuna (in descending order, Japan, Taiwan, Indonesia, Spain, Korea, United States, Philippines, Mexico, France, and Ecuador).[11]

The rise, fall, then rise again of tuna sales occurred over approximately a three-year period, from about 1970 to 1973. The swordfish industry, on the other hand, would struggle for five more years, as the mercury levels found in this fish were higher than those in tuna. For fears to be allayed, the swordfish industry, too, continued to try to prove that the amounts of methylmercury found in its fish were safe to consume, and what better place to find willing volunteers than a place where the subjects were employed by the fishing industry in question? For this purpose, Peru seemed a natural. One of the largest swordfish fisheries in Latin America at the time was that of Peruvians off the country's northern coast. By 1950 catches amounted to as much as seven thousand tons, though they saw a significant decline in the 1990s.[12]

In Peru there were two studies, both conducted by the University of Rochester. The first was of adults and was reported initially at the Spanish mint in 1974. It had the same funding as the Samoan study, including the Tuna Research Foundation. Researchers compared two fishing communities on the north coast, Mancora and Cancas, to the agricultural village of Morropon, fifty kilometers from Mancora, in the period 1972–1985. The second study was one of infant-mother pairs drawn from the same areas. To get data on consumption patterns, dieticians in the adult study questioned the housewife from each family concerning diet and the daily intake of fish, with "particular attention to swordfish."[13] Neurologists were to pay special attention to sensations around the mouth and limbs but did not conduct specific psychological testing. The Spanish-speaking physician conducting the medical history was instructed to be alert to any symptoms of methylmercury intoxication.

The 1974 report did not address symptoms other than the overt ones, such as paresthesia, hearing loss, tunnel vision, impairment of walking or movement of the limbs, and trouble speaking.[14]

Since David Marsh, John Crispin-Smith, and other members of the Rochester team were essentially looking only for symptoms of methylmercury intoxication, which typically occur at much higher levels than what these populations were exposed to, it appears the symptom range for diagnosis in the Peru study of adults was limited. The Peruvian physicians would likely overlook potentially significant complaints that the Rochester group had been identifying as insignificant.

In 1980, the 1974 Peru paper was finally published in a peer-reviewed journal. Results were given for 190 subjects from the fishing villages and 93 from the agricultural villages. In the fishing villages, the average blood methylmercury level was 82 mcg/l, with a range of 11–275 mcg/l. The most common complaint was limb paresthesia (29.5%), followed by impaired vision (7.9%), backache (6.8%), and dizziness (5.3%).

As for the farmers, their average methylmercury level was 9.9 mcg/l, with a range of 3.3–25.1 mcg/l. They complained of paresthesia (49.5%), headache (16.1%), abdominal discomfort (11.8%), nervousness (10.8%), dizziness (8.6%), backache (7.5%), and leg cramps or pain (6.5%). Despite these symptoms at comparatively low mercury exposure levels, the conclusion was that the "Peruvian population . . . appears similar to the few others that have been studied in showing no apparent ill effects from ingestion of considerable quantities of methylmercury from ocean fish."[15]

Not only were a number of the symptoms serious, however, but the comparison of the two groups was flawed. The farmers were not an adequate control group—they had mercury in their blood. In other words, the researchers compared the somewhat exposed to the more exposed. A statistical significance of symptoms would be less likely with such a comparison.

The incidence of paresthesia in both these populations seemed extraordinary to me. I looked at the *Physician's Desk Reference* and randomly selected the drug Zofran (GlaxoSmithKline) to look at the clinical trial for the incidence of paresthesia in the otherwise healthy placebo group. Only about 1 percent complained of it. As for the incidence of this symptom in the general population, many causes are known, such as multiple sclerosis, toxic substances, metabolic disorders, vitamin deficiencies and overdoses, and many others. Perhaps you could say that everyone has experienced this symptom transiently after sitting in a position that caused a limb to "fall asleep." I have been practicing medicine for seventeen years, and it is not a common symptom, transient episodes aside. I would estimate it as less than 2 percent for my patient population.

The most common symptoms I see in my patient population exposed to methylmercury, and the symptoms seen in other types of mercury toxicities, were not asked about. These are insomnia, fatigue, hair loss, depression, agitation or other personality change, memory loss, trouble thinking, trouble with word finding, trouble performing complex tasks, trouble with concentration, metallic taste in the mouth, muscle pain, fainting or feeling faint, excessive salivation, and excessive sweating. The authors did, however, ask if the subjects had a poor memory, headache, generalized weakness, arm pain, or leg pain.

Research on Peruvian mothers and infants was not published until 1995. Funding then was listed as from the National Oceanic and Atmospheric Administration (NOAA), the National Fisheries Institute, and the Tuna Research Foundation. The same Rochester neurologists performed exams in the Peru study as in the Iraq and Samoan studies. After looking at basic parameters such as whether the infants sat, stood, walked, and talked at appropriate stages of development and checking for movement abnormalities, retarded speech, and mental retardation, their conclusion again was that there was no increase in the frequency of neurodevelopmental abnormalities in early childhood. There was no indication of extensive neurodevelopmental testing, however, and details of methods of data collection were lacking.[16]

In studies of symptoms based mainly on self-report of subjective criteria, it's important to consider what cultural factors or immediate circumstances might play a role in what is reported. In Peru, several such complicating factors were potentially of great importance but were not addressed in the Rochester group's mercury papers.

First, what was the potential role of coca leaves in mediating the adult population's experience of mercury-related symptoms? Peru was the largest producer of coca leaves in the world, and the Andean tradition of chewing coca leaves is centuries old. People use the leaves in rituals and for easing hunger, as protection against cold in the high Andean altitudes, and to create a sense of well-being. Seventy distinct folk medicines are based on coca leaves, and more than 80 percent of the rural high Andean population use the coca leaf for some form of health care.[17] Coca use is not confined to Andean areas but is also found in lower-elevation agricultural areas, in cities, and in coastal regions.

Although coca can ease the ache of hard labor, maybe even the pain of mercury, it was certainly curious that the farmers had a higher incidence of paresthesias than the fishermen. The possible answer could be in what the farmers were growing and where they were growing it. Coca growers prefer to grow the plants at higher altitudes because coca plants grown there have been found to contain a higher percentage of the cocaine alkaloid than those grown at lower altitudes. A scientific study of Peru residents published in 2002 demonstrated that the low oxygen levels experienced at high elevations are highly correlated with paresthesias, especially if one is susceptible to mountain sickness.[18] Coca farmers may be laboring at high elevations, which could lead to a higher incidence of paresthesias compared to the fishermen at sea level. Extent of exposure to agricultural pesticides and chemicals also was not considered in the study, as some agricultural chemicals can cause neurological symptoms such as paresthesia, nervousness, and abdominal discomfort, of which the farmers complained in a higher percentage than did people living in the fishing villages.

The most important omission in the Peruvian studies was information on whether some of the subjects had a history of working in or living near the country's mercury mines, which would have exposed them to elemental mercury. In the adult study, the authors tested for methylmercury but not for total mercury levels.[19] This would be important to note, since the "total" mercury level would be the methylmercury plus any inorganic or elemental mercury, as would be picked up in mercury mining. The researchers again concluded, "No individual was identified with symptoms or signs that could be attributed to methylmercury intoxication."[20]

In the Peru and Samoa studies, only looking for overt symptoms, as defined by the Iraq study by the Rochester group, would certainly keep the idea alive that no one is affected by consuming methylmercury at these lower exposure levels. It appears these researchers were convincing, as physicians, public health officials, current employees of the FDA, nongovernment groups, journalists, and many others still feel there were adequate studies to prove this notion. The symptom profile of what constituted mercury toxicity, including the level of exposure at which symptoms occurred, was being laid down by a group of researchers that received funding not just from government agencies, but also concerned industry groups. When a potentially misleading "signs and symptoms" profile of a syndrome as complex as mercury toxicity becomes established in the scientific literature, it can take decades to correct. But there was to be still more to the story.

CHAPTER 15

The Political Realm of
Seychelles versus Faroes

IN 2003, AFTER I AND MY FISH-EATING PATIENTS had been making
headlines, I received a call from a man who claimed to be a physician representing a group of ocean fishermen who were concerned
about my study. He explained that he had "a group of guys" who were
commercial fishermen who just could not believe that a person could
get such elevated mercury levels in their blood from consuming commercial fish. His "guys" wanted to show everyone this was not true by
testing their own blood. They consumed a lot of fish, he had determined, and thought they would be ideal for this endeavor. I thought to
myself, what an interesting strategy—consuming your own product,
known to have mercury, and then testing yourself for it. After the blood
levels kept coming in elevated, a person who attends fisheries-related
conventions told me, they abandoned the project. But this stuck in my
mind, that the fishing industry seemed to have a general strategy to
prove that mercury in fish is harmless. Surely it was one reason that the
Tuna Foundation kept reappearing as a funder of selected research.
The American Samoa and Peru fishermen and their families were willing to help in this endeavor, it seemed. Were they doing it out of concern for their health, company loyalty, or simply fear of losing their
livelihood? One can only wonder.

Despite the favorable outcome for the fishing industry in the
Anderson trial, there remained an area where the industry was still vulnerable: determinations of the minimum dose of mercury that would
result in brain damage for a developing fetus. In the 1980s a study was
conducted, again by Thomas Clarkson and his team, of another
unique population, this time to examine the mercury effects on early

development in the Republic of Seychelles. In the same decade, another independent long-term project was begun in the Faroe Islands of Denmark on the effects of mercury toxicity and the health of children, this one led by Philippe Grandjean, a professor at Harvard University and the University of Southern Denmark.

It is the Faroes study that the EPA relied on to set its current standards for methylmercury in fish consumption, and it is the Seychelles study that the industry relies on as a counter. The FDA still has not fully embraced either. If it did embrace the former, the action level for methylmercury in fish would most likely need to be lowered back to 0.5 mcg/g and the warnings of mercury's dangers made more explicit.

The Faroes are made up of eighteen islands, population about 45,000, covering an area of 1,400 square kilometers (slightly less than 550 square miles) in the North Atlantic. The people are a self-governing part of the Kingdom of Denmark, a country where, overall, fisheries and agriculture account for less than 3 percent of the GDP. The inclusion of whale meat and fish in the diet of the Faroese apparently depended on local availability and personal preferences and not on socioeconomic factors such as family income. Except for food from the sea and lamb, potatoes, and some dairy products, most food was imported from mainland Europe. In the Faroes economy, fishing is a major contributor, especially in the form of farmed salmon (a fish that contains very little mercury), but fishing constitutes a small part of the Kingdom of Denmark's economy. According to one report, "The [Faroes] economy is dependent upon fishery exports for nearly 97 percent of the nation's total foreign exchange earnings. In recent years, the catch of traditional species of cod, haddock, and whiting has declined, making fish farming a valuable source of future export earnings." Interestingly, fish farms in the Faroes were privately owned by individual farmers, not by the government or large corporations.[1]

Philippe Grandjean began his studies in 1986 and has been funded over the years by the U.S. National Institute of Environmental Health Sciences, the European Commission, United Nations University, the Danish Medical Research Council, the Dannin Foundation, U.S. FDA, EPA, and the Nissan Science Foundation. Grandjean compared exposed individuals to a control population that was significantly less exposed, on mercury-relevant tests, in order to obtain a threshold level where adverse effects occurred in the study subjects. The initial mercury testing consisted of blood samples taken from the baby's umbilical cord at birth. This was thought to be a good measure of exposure during pregnancy, as methylmercury freely crosses the placenta, the baby's blood binds mercury stronger than the mother's blood, and a baby does not rid himself or herself of mercury. Grandjean's team administered a battery of neuropsychiatric tests as the children grew older, and reports were published after tests were completed at ages seven and fourteen. These examinations consisted of a medical history and questionnaire that encompassed the mother and child, a physical exam, and a series of intelligence and neurobehavioral tests.[2] The median cord blood mercury was found to be five times higher in the exposed subjects compared to the controls (59.0 mcg/l vs. 11.9 mcg/l), Grandjean found. (The mothers' median hair mercury level was 12.5 mcg/g for the study subjects and 1.8 mcg/g for the controls. This would correspond to about 50.0 mcg/l and 8.0 mcg/l in blood, respectively.)[3] A control population that had no measurable mercury again would have been ideal for teasing out subtle neurological differences between the two groups, but may not have been possible to assemble in this instance.

Statistically significant adverse effects occurred at cord blood levels of 58 mcg/l and up. In order to calculate a dose for mercury below which there would be no statistically significant effects on children, the researchers calculated in an uncertainty factor (previously known as a safety factor) of ten. This uncertainty factor took into consideration the variability of individuals, circumstances, and differences in mercury metabolism between individuals, so that even the most sensitive individuals would be protected, should this level be reached. Grandjean and his colleagues concluded that one should keep one's blood mercury level less than 5.8 mcg/l.[4] This corresponds to the EPA's reference dose of less than 0.1 mcg/kg body weight a day. For a 132-pound (60-kilogram) person, this would mean consuming less than 6 mcg of mercury per day. The importance of determining the minimum-effect level rose even more when it was discovered that newborns can have a level of mercury two to three times higher than their mothers, since the infant cannot rid itself of it until after birth. Arguments over the need for even stricter guidelines are ongoing.[5]

In the Faroes study, the mercury-exposed group in infancy showed mild decrements compared to the control group in the areas of motor function, language, and memory. At seven and fourteen years of age, slowing of brain stem functions, such as auditory reaction times to a stimuli, correlated with methylmercury exposure that occurred in utero. Some of these effects appear to be permanent, as they continued at age fourteen.[6]

The major criticism from industry researchers of the Faroes study was that some subjects ate some whale meat and farmed salmon, which would expose them to polychlorinated biphenyl compounds (PCBs) and that could make difficult the analysis of their symptoms. PCBs are mixtures of 209 manmade chlorinated compounds that were used to make substances such as coolants, lubricants, capacitors, and electrical insulation. Their use is now banned in the United States and many other countries because of evidence that they cause cancer, disrupt the endocrine system, and may damage the developing brain. Dr. Grandjean and his team concluded that omega-3 fatty acid concentrations, considered beneficial, and the PCB concentrations, considered harmful, when analyzed together may have caused them to underestimate the toxic effects of mercury.[7] Regardless, Dr. Grandjean's study on mercury exposure is ongoing, and only time will tell if any other effects become evident in the children's lives that can be linked to methylmercury exposure in utero.

As for the fish industry, it still needed to prove that methylmercury exposure from eating mercury-laden fish high in the food chain was safe. The credit for finding a willing group to study for this purpose goes to the Tropical Products Institute (TPI), a London food-based company that was involved in the processing and marketing of foodstuffs to include fish. In 1981, A. D. Matthews of TPI began a survey in the Seychelles on people's fish intake, their mercury levels, and the mercury content of fish caught in their waters. In the initial survey of mercury levels in fishermen and their wives and babies in the Republic of the

Seychelles, published in 1983, Matthews found them to be elevated compared to populations in other parts of the world and suggested that a more detailed study was needed.[8]

Here was another population of fishermen and their wives that was exposed to methylmercury through fish consumption and that, Matthews suggested, would volunteer for a study to tell whether methylmercury in fish was harmful. The fishing industry now had to decide whether studying this population would be worth the effort. If adverse effects were found, the fishing industry would suffer; if no effects were found, it could delay and perhaps stop any further regulation or policy making when it came to mercury and fish, and perhaps even regulation on mercury pollution as a whole. Finding no harm could bring more tuna boats to the country, and thus strengthen the economy and improve residents' lives. But, with more environmental regulations and pollution control orders on mercury in various countries creeping up, more funding would have to come from other interested parties for this task. As mentioned in earlier chapters, the power industry's lobbying group, Electric Power Research Institute, funded some of the Seychelles study. The fishing industry did, as well, as did the governments of the Seychelles and the United States. This gave the appearance of a "we're in this together" type of arrangement. The EPA was about to crack down on pollution in general in the mid-1980s, and just how long the polluting industries could keep mercury off the list of harmful agents depended on the fishing industry's ability to prove there was no harm from exposure through the fish that were allegedly contaminated by the polluting industries.

Because the Tropical Products Institute was instrumental in initiating the Seychelles Child Development Study, the Rochester researchers give 1981 as the official start date in some scientific papers and 1983 in others. Enrollment for the "pilot" study (the initial survey to see if a major study should be undertaken) took place in 1987–1988, while the main cohort was enrolled in 1989. In essence, one could say there were two pilot surveys, as Matthews conducted the first, which led the Rochester researchers to the second. In Rochester's pilot study, the median mercury level in the mothers' hair was 6.6 mcg/g, with a range of 0.59–36.4 mcg/g. Of the 789 mothers, 140 had levels greater than 12 mcg/g (approximately 48 mcg/l blood). The pilot study consisted of a questionnaire, followed by a physical exam, then a basic neurological exam and a variety of tests of children's development before the age of two. The researchers concluded, "The present study did find an association between fetal mercury exposure in the low ranges tested in developmental but not neurological end-points during the first two years of life." In other words, the initial study begun by the Rochester group did show some adverse develop-mental effects that were related to mercury exposure. This was not published, though, until 1995.[9]

In 2000, a published report appeared describing a select group of eighty-seven children from the pilot cohort who were given a battery of tests at the age of nine. The researchers found that on some tests, higher mercury levels were actually associated with a better perform-ance, although on one test performance was worse. They concluded that no adverse effects from methylmercury could be confirmed—at least not among these individuals selected for testing later in child-hood.[10]

In 1995, many reports appeared in one volume of the journal *Neu-rotoxicology* on mercury and the Seychelles children. The main study consisted of 740 new infant-mother pairs in which the children were followed through six and a half months of age. Instead of cord blood mercury as tested in the Faroes, the researchers tested the moth-ers' hair mercury level before, during or after they gave birth. The median for the mothers' hair mercury level listed was 5.9 mcg/g. The researchers concluded that no neurodevelopmental effects related to fetal mercury exposure could be demonstrated in the young children, though they cautioned that further studies at later ages might detect developmental differences.[11]

By 2003, the Seychelles Child Development Study main cohort was tested at about nine years of age. Boys in the study showed a decreased performance on a pegboard test using their nondominant hand as mer-cury exposure increased. It was also reported that the study subjects had a better score on the hyperactivity index with higher mercury exposure levels. Both outcomes were thought to be due to chance; therefore, the authors concluded, "These data do not support the hypothesis that there is a neurodevelopmental risk from prenatal MeHg [methylmercury] exposure resulting solely from ocean fish consumption."[12]

In the Seychelles Child Development Study, the benchmark dose (the dose at which significant effects occur) was calculated, using the mothers' hair mercury level at the birth of the child, and was determined to be 25 mcg/g.[13] This would mean that the level of mercury in the mothers' blood was in the ballpark of 100 mcg/l. Although the researchers concluded no effects, they determined a benchmark through extrapolation that was only twice that of the Faroes study.

The Seychelles island community on which the study took place was only 150 square kilometers in area and had only one hospital and twelve clinics. Enrollment of the children was done by Seychellois research nurses,[14] on Mahé who contacted the families through the network of maternal and child health and offered participation in the study to all mothers listed in the logbooks. One scientific report stated, "No data were collected concerning reasons that mothers did not bring their child for examination. 'Informally,' these were reported to include families who were not contacted, did not understand the study, had conflicting responsibilities, did not want their child examined, or were superstitious about having hair taken from themselves or their child. This translated to including 50 percent of all live births in the Republic of Seychelles during the enrollment period into the study."[15]

In the main study, the senior research nurse and two clinical nurses assigned by the Seychelles government from the Ministry of Health worked full-time with the primary investigators. They claimed that clinicians, mothers, and other observers, in both Seychelles and Rochester, were unable to influence the responses on the basis of exposure levels because they wouldn't have known those levels.[16] But calculations could be done to estimate a person's load and subsequent mercury level, as the average mercury levels in the fish consumed had been determined by Matthews, and dietary surveys were asked of the mothers prior to the testing of the children.

A more in-depth look at the Seychelles found a conflict of interest that I had not read about in the scientific papers, and that needs to be considered if one is to apply their study results for use in clinical practice. During the years of the study, the country of Seychelles was also creating a tuna empire, which could have influenced how residents and researchers saw the issues surrounding mercury.

The Republic of Seychelles is a sovereign nation that consists of 115 islands in the Indian Ocean. The people are predominantly African and European in origin, and a French and English Creole dialect is the main language spoken at home. Of the two main islands, Mahé and Prasin, the study took place on Mahé, an island only 150 square kilometers large but containing 90 percent of the population—about 67,000 people during the Seychelles Child Development Study.[17] In the nation's economy, exports played a substantial role, and among those, canned tuna, frozen and fresh fish, frozen prawns, and cinnamon bark led the list.[18] According to a 1999 survey conducted by the International Trade Centre (ITC), the export of fish and fish products accounted for more than 97 percent of the Seychelles domestic export for the year 1998 (excluding tourism). In 1998, fishing and fisheries-related activities contributed about 22 percent of gross domestic product but 50 percent of foreign exchange earnings.[19]

There were only four firms in the Seychelles engaged in the export of fish products, according to this report. The first was Indian Ocean Tuna Ltd., formed in 1987, the sole company engaged in tuna canning in Seychelles and the nation's largest employer. In 1995 the American food company H.J. Heinz acquired 60 percent of the shares of Indian Ocean Tuna, and it became a joint venture between the Seychelles government and Heinz. The second and third companies were Sea Harvest (Pty) Ltd. and Oceana Fisheries Company Ltd., each formed in 1995 and engaged in long-lining for tuna and swordfish, as well as bottom fishing, and in the purchase and export of fresh and frozen fish. The fourth company was the Seychelles Marketing Board. Formed in 1984, it was one of the biggest companies in the Seychelles and was engaged in a wide range of commercial activities, including the production and export of black tiger prawns.[20]

During the years of the Seychelles Child Development Study, the country's tuna industry was booming. When the Seychelles tuna canning company was set up in 1987, it had a capacity of 50 metric tons per day. After its acquisition by Heinz in 1995, the plant's production capacity grew to reach 250 metric tons per day by 1998. The volume of canned tuna exported grew by almost 250 percent in that period, and its value increased from US$18.4 million to $78.6 million. Heinz, which sold its canned tuna under the labels StarKist in the United States and John West in Europe, sold its interest to Del Monte Foods in 2002.[21]

By 2001, exports of canned tuna alone accounted for 91 percent of the total fish exports and 87 percent of the Seychelles visible export. The Seychelles' facility was the second-largest tuna cannery in the world after StarKist Samoa. "Reduced production," one report concluded, "would have catastrophic results for a small island community."[22]

StarKist/Heinz and the Seychelles government had a stake in the outcome of the study, that is certain, just as StarKist did in American Samoa. The influence, if any, that the fishing industry had on the subjects or on the researchers as they studied methylmercury in a nation highly dependent on the fishing industry would be difficult to determine without declaration by those involved. The influence that the researchers had on the economy of the tuna industry was certainly a positive one. Hopefully, the people of the Seychelles benefited from their hard labor in the tuna canning industry.[23]

By 2006, new statistical calculations were published on the Seychelles Child Development Study, with Clarkson as an author. I was surprised that in the discussion section, the authors quoted a Clarkson paper that said the WHO Iraqi data had estimated a no-observable-adverse-effect level (NOAEL or NOEL) of 10–20 ppm (mcg/g) in hair.[24] I consulted with Dr. Grandjean and asked if the Iraqi data derived a no-adverse-effect level. He responded, "You can't derive a no-observable-effect level from epidemiologic data."[25]

This is what was so confusing to the public and the physicians, and anyone else looking at the papers. Saying a NOEL was determined or estimated implied that a mercury level in the human body had been found below which no symptoms were related to mercury. But that was never true, because researchers simply had not done that type of study; at least not one that was published that I could find. They can guess, extrapolate, or just make one up, but an actual study that would ascertain a true no-effect level for humans has not been done.

In this 2006 paper on the Seychelles Child Development Study, the researchers concluded that at the nine-year follow-up, their benchmark mercury concentration (the concentration at which adverse effects begin to occur) was 20 mcg/g in the mothers' hair (about 80 mcg/l blood) and was slightly lower than what they had calculated before. This benchmark was moving closer to what the Faroes study determined (58 mcg/l cord blood). Even so, they concluded that although they "were not aware of any evidence to suggest that subtle differences in cognitive and motor performance reported in relation to prenatal methylmercury exposure impaired an individual child's overall ability to function . . . it has been argued that the societal implications of such subtle changes, especially on IQ, may be important for a population."[26]

Both the Faroes blood benchmark of 58 mcg/l and the Seychelles one of 80 mcg/l are far lower than the 400 mcg/l that was used to set— apparently in stone—the current FDA action level in fish at 1 mcg/g. Now that there is an indication that methylmercury in fish can cause harm at these levels, the polluting industries will have a more difficult time fending off regulation. Or will they?

CHAPTER 16

The Mercury Study Report

OVER RECENT DECADES, while the fishing industry was pushing back against FDA policy, many other groups were wondering where all the mercury was coming from in the first place. It seemed a complicated matter, but someone needed to show congressional leaders what to make of it all. And the issue extends far beyond the boundaries of the United States. Developing standards for mercury was a high-stakes game with a lot of money to be gained or lost, to say nothing of the human well-being at risk from mercury poisoning.

Not only had large conglomerate food corporations already suffered economic loss by the wrath generated by fears of mercury contamination in the early 1970s, entire nations were dependent on the fishing industry as their source of income and relied on fish as a good source of healthful protein. With more than five thousand tons of mercury bellowing into the air annually worldwide, we cannot continue to allow industry to proceed as if its pollution causes no harm to the environment just because fishermen and their families appear to have an apparent immunity to the toxic effects of methylmercury. In the mix is the cost of mercury pollution in industrial waste in water, soil, and air; air pollution caused by mercury emissions from coal-burning power plants; mercury in commonly used products such as latex paint and mercury/silver dental amalgams; ethylmercury in the common preservative thimerosal in vaccines; mercury batteries, switches, computers— a tangle of issues difficult for anyone to sort out.

During the quest for the human effects of mercury toxicity in the 1970s and 1980s, many other issues were on the grill. Mercury pollution was becoming an ever greater concern in the United States, as environmentalists and various nongovernment organizations weighed in. By 1990, coal-burning power companies were feeling the pressure to reduce mercury emissions in the wake of passage of the Clean Air Act of 1986. This act was an extensive 466-page call not only for clean air, but also for the study of all types of airborne pollution known at the time and their effects on humans and the ecosystem. The act also called for grants for support of air pollution planning and control programs. Each state was to come up with a plan for reducing its ambient air pollutants. Federal facilities would also have to find better ways to control emissions.

The Clean Air Act Amendments of 1990 subsequently ordered the EPA to study and report in four years on mercury emissions from electric utility steam-generating units, municipal waste combustion units, and other sources. The EPA was to consider the rate and mass of such emissions, the health and environmental effects, technologies available to control such emissions, and the costs of such technologies. The National Institute of Environmental Health Sciences (NIEHS) was ordered to conduct and transmit to Congress within three years a study to determine the threshold for mercury concentrations in tissue of fish that may be consumed (including consumption by sensitive populations) without adverse effects to public health.[1]

As the finger pointing began on who was most responsible for polluting the air, water, and subsequently the fish, the power companies who burned coal that emitted mercury into the air began digging in their heels. Coal contains mercury naturally, and when it is burned, mercury is released into the air. Some types of coal, such as lignite, emit higher amounts of mercury than others. From the air, mercury settles not only over the land but also in the waterways, where it is absorbed by bacteria in soil and water and transformed into methylmercury, the more dangerous mercury compound. The plankton eat the bacteria, the fish eat the plankton, the bigger fish eat the smaller fish, and the problem becomes amplified through the food chain.

In the midst of this controversy over coal-fired power plants, Thomas Clarkson again found his way to the scene. In 1991, a paper that was written by Clarkson and William Fitzgerald and partially funded by the power company lobby the Electric Power Research

Institute, weighed in on the issue of mercury emissions from power companies: "It is strikingly evident that modest increases in atmospheric mercury loading could lead directly to elevated levels in fish stock," it said. And the article continued: "It is doubtful, given the experimental limitations in many recent studies, that the temporal pattern for mercury emissions, for background atmospheric mercury concentrations, and for changes in mercury depositional fluxes has been identified."[2] In other words, there is mercury in the air, but as described in the paper even that seems to be a mystery. The mercury is getting into the water, and may even be getting into the fish, but the authors could not say for sure where all the mercury found in the fish was coming from, as it might not be the power companies causing the problem. They concluded that there was a "great need for an extensive study on a fish-eating population covering the range of methylmercury intakes associated with the lowest effect levels estimated from the Iraq outbreak."[3]

At that time, the Faroes study had already begun, as well as the Seychelles Child Development Study. But their results would not be published until 1997 and 1995, respectively. If methylmercury in fish caused harm, the next step for the coal-fired power companies would be to say that it was not their mercury that was in the fish. The Seychelles study would be what industry was counting on, as evidence from the Faroes study from Harvard and Denmark and a report from the EPA were bearing down on them. They were all going to try to tell us how much pollution our environment and health could take.

The *Mercury Study Report to Congress* was led by an EPA scientist by the name of Martha Keating. She was the project director and a principal author of the report. Kathryn Mahaffey of EPA joined the project in 1993. In my interviews with Keating and Mahaffey, conducted independently of one another, they noted that although the report was due in 1994, it was not completed until 1995. It was then further delayed by the Office of Management and Budget (OMB) under the Clinton administration. According to Keating, Vice President Al Gore told her the delay was because the Seychelles mercury study was soon to be released, and industry, the FDA, members of Congress, and other interest groups wanted the Seychelles study to be heard before policy was to be made.

The Alaskan senators were especially concerned, according to Keating, as the largest fishing corporation in the United States was Arctic Alaska Fisheries, and they apparently felt that the Alaskan economy could be adversely affected by the report if the amount of mercury allowed in fish was further regulated.

According to Mahaffey, the OMB held up the progress of the report after being influenced by lobbyists from the fishing and power plant industries. She felt the OMB was "unduly harsh" in its criticism. The report went through more than 120 reviewers, Mahaffey said, which was atypical at that time. Letters of opposition and editing out of important facts were plentiful. One important graph that OMB demanded be removed, and subsequently was, concerned mercury and fish consumption risk. Another removed item was an estimate by the report's authors that 7 percent to 10 percent of the U.S. population was at risk of overexposure to mercury—enough to pose harm. OMB would not approve the estimate and demanded that it be revised to 1 percent to 3 percent. Mahaffey and Keating were successful in keeping in a much protested statement that high-end consumers not limited by income who consume a large portion of their dietary protein from fish—especially if they chose large predators such as swordfish, sea bass, and the like—would be at risk for toxic exposure to mercury.

The report did conclude, though, that coal-fired power plants accounted for the largest amount of mercury emissions in the air. It also concluded that people should keep their blood mercury levels below 4 to 5 mcg/l in order to protect the developing fetus, infants, small children, and exposure over a lifetime. In the end, the report went without some important information, as the OMB, advisory committees that contained industry representatives, and the Rochester researchers opposed many findings and conclusions—on what grounds is not clear, as those opposition letters were never published.[4]

Evidence of the Alaskan interest in the matter was confirmed by a letter from Alaska's Division of Public Health, which was published in *Science*. "Severely limiting the consumption of fish and seafood may do more harm than good by reducing the consumption of foods with health benefits and by increasing the consumption of alternative foods that have potential health risks," the authors of the letter argued. "For populations that rely heavily on subsistence fishing, restrictive fish consumption advisories could damage the social, economic, and personal well-being of entire villages. . . . In Canada, the general health status of subsistence populations worsened after the social, economic, lifestyle, and dietary changes associated with fish consumption advisories."[5]

The authors of the letter failed to mention that the Ojibway, the Canadian population to whom they were referring, were affected by consuming fish from an unfortunate industrial poisoning and not from the ocean fishing industry. Although it's true that the Indians' economy evaporated, their health was compromised as well. The authors' statements did not appear to take a protective approach for the above-average fish consumer. Nor did they distinguish between the very high mercury content in the polluted lakes and the elevated mercury levels in ocean fish, though one would think it would have been in their best interest to separate themselves from the overt pollution problem that had occurred in Canada. Furthermore, the letter made the Alaska Division of Public Health seem little concerned with the region's at-risk subpopulations whose members consumed an inordinate amount of mercury. Thomas Clarkson and his Rochester group also wrote a letter to the editor of *Science*, the following month, agreeing with the Alaska Public Health Division's charge.[6]

In looking into the scientific studies that were available to the EPA scientists, Dr. Grandjean's first report on his Faroes study was published in 1997 and concluded that there were adverse health effects from the consumption of methylmercury in fish. The results from the Seychelles Child Development Study, published in 1995, which showed no adverse effects to children, was also considered. Still, the release of the *Mercury Study Report* was impeded by industry groups and lobbyists as they did not agree that mercury was harmful at the levels seen in the Faroes study. The Natural Resources Defense Council and the Sierra Club began a legal battle to have the EPA's report released and objected to the government's stalling.

The *Mercury Study Report to Congress* was finally released in December 1997. Because a study that shows no effects from a drug or toxicant cannot negate a study that shows effects, the Faroes reference dose (RfD) (a dose of mercury under which no harm is expected) was used to set the EPA's methylmercury consumption guidelines. This RfD included the uncertainty factor of ten, formally known in the Anderson trial as the "safety factor." After the report became public, Congress required the EPA to fund the National Academy of Sciences (NAS) to review the literature and the RfD. In 2000, the NAS came out in support of the EPA's RfD: 0.1 mcg/kg body weight/day. A person consuming this amount of mercury would have an estimated blood level of 4–5 mcg/l. Mercury was subsequently added to the list of toxicants regulated under the Clean Air Act on December 20, 2000.[7]

With that confirmation of the EPA's RfD for mercury, not only the fishing industry but also the coal-burning power plants were threatened. Fishing, coal mining, and coal-fired power plant operations might be critical industries for the health of the U.S. economy, but the *Mercury Study Report* implicated coal-burning power plants as the largest contributor to mercury pollution in the air.

When it comes to fish, the EPA therefore had a clear RfD for mercury, but the EPA gives advisories only for noncommercial fish. The FDA is the agency that gives advisories for commercial fish, and it had already lost a major battle in the 1977 Anderson trial in trying to enforce its rules on the amount of methylmercury allowed in fish and what was considered safe. The FDA had issued a fish advisory in conjunction with the EPA's in 2006, as we've seen, but only for infants, small children, pregnant women, and women of reproductive age. For others, the FDA still allowed mercury in fish to be consumed at a level that would place a consumer over the EPA's recommended maximum.

Because the FDA's action level for fish is still at 1 mcg/g, it does not protect those who consume the higher-mercury-content fish, nor those who consume a higher quantity of fish. In other words, the amount of mercury allowed in fish can result in too high a dose for some individuals. A person who chooses fish such as the large tunas, sea bass, orange roughy, and large halibut on a regular basis could be within the

FDA's consumption guidelines—twice a week consumption—but over the EPA's mercury level guideline. This was the situation of many of my patients, as some consumed fish only twice a week but had mercury levels several times over 5 mcg/l.

In looking at the literature, there was more to read about than just the fetal effects. Mercury studies on adults showed that there was a correlation between elevated mercury levels from fish consumption and heart attack and carotid artery disease at a level near the EPA's safe level. In one ongoing study on Finnish men, first reported in 1995, the authors concluded that consumption of mercury only twice that of the RfD not only could negate the good effects of omega-3 fatty acids in fish but could double your risk of heart attack, as well. These new findings were a devastating blow to those who had been pushing omega-3 fatty acids in the form of fish for cardiac health.[8]

But leave it to StarKist to find a novel way to advertise the good virtues of fish. The American Heart Association's (AHA's) "Heart Healthy" label that is on so many food items today became established in 1995, after about seven years of debates with the FDA and the food industry. StarKist claims to be the first tuna certified by the AHA.[9]

The FDA wanted to encourage the American population to consume more fish. But to discourage those individuals who already consumed a lot of mercury, the agency took what it referred to as a "nuanced," or "targeted" approach, in which only reproductive or nursing females and infants and small children were given warning of mercury's danger. The message, then, involved telling the public that mercury was okay to consume while at the same time saying it could be harmful to their health. The targeted, nuanced approach also insinuated to the rest of the public that the high-end consumption pattern was not harmful unless you happened to be very young, pregnant, or nursing.

Not disclosing a contaminant that could damage your health would be unthinkable if the said poison was added in the process of making a food—if that food was, in other words, "adulterated." The Anderson case ensured that fish was not considered adulterated until its mercury content was over 1 mcg/g. This allowed the food industry to avoid placing labels on fish. If you had to declare the contaminants in all food on labels, much as is now done for ingredients, almost every food item would have a warning. Substances such as caffeine, saturated fat, and now even transfat (when it's more than 0.5 grams) are declared in the ingredients of food and beverage items, but mercury has not been.

The food industry is packed with lobbyists, lawyers, executives, and word sleuths. They often support multiple candidates and political parties to cover all their bases. The mercury saga is but one example of how the political wrangling and positioning works. Let's take a look at how President William Jefferson Clinton dealt with the *Mercury Study Report to Congress* in the face of his donors.[10]

Recalling his early days in Arkansas in the 1970s, Bill Clinton said in his memoir, "The local political hangout was Billie Schneider's Steakhouse on Highway 71. . . . All the local politicos hung out in her place, including Don Tyson and Don Tyson's lawyer, Jim Blair, a 6-foot five-inch idiosyncratic genius who would become one of my closest friends." When he spoke of Jim Blair's wife, Diane, he said, "Diane and Hillary became more than friends; they were soul mates."[11]

Don Tyson, a significant donator to Clinton's political campaigns, was the founder of the Arkansas-based poultry conglomerate Tyson foods and was influential in directing Clinton on several issues that affected the Tyson food business.[12] In 1992, while the *Mercury Study Report* was under way, Tyson Foods bought the largest fishery in the United States, Arctic Alaska Fisheries, Inc., and Louis Kemp seafood. Don Tyson, therefore, had a large stake in the outcome of any mercury studies and would want his interests protected. It was the Alaskans who, by state, had the biggest voice opposing any further regulation when it came to mercury in fish, and had influence on delaying the release of the report.[13]

Despite the *Mercury Study Report*'s call to consume less in the way of mercury and to reduce mercury pollution and opposition to the EPA report from Alaskan politicians, Alaska ironically went on to develop a significant fishery economy and now is leading the world in sustainable fishery practices. With the rising awareness of fish contaminants such as mercury and PCBs, Alaskan fish has become even more in demand, as the public perceives Alaska's waters and the fish that swim in them to be less influenced by human industrial contamination. Alaskan inland waters are by no means pristine, though. A report released in the year 2000 from a conservation group stated that Alaska had more than two thousand contaminated sites and six Superfund sites. Most of the pollution came from the military, industry, oil and gas development, and mining, as well as toxic releases from Russia and Asia. Efforts to monitor the contaminants in fish are ongoing.[14]

Politicians have to weigh the pros and cons not only on the issues at hand, but also on how their positions on those issues will affect their political futures. Their conflicts of interest are bound to surface, as politicians represent many constituents. But when policy decisions involve public health, avoiding conflicts of interest is particularly crucial. Making money at the expense of someone's health is inexcusable. Therefore, as more environmental issues arise that involve the health of living beings and the economy, a more open forum will need to be instituted. People need to make their own decisions based on sound information. In the age of the Internet, the information jet stream allows for more information to be obtained, but it is only valuable to the extent that researchers, government agencies, nongovernment agencies, industry, and other commentators do the best they can to give accurate information.

Although the *Mercury Study Report* sparked heavy discussion on both sides, and its publication was delayed for at least two years, the Clinton administration, Tyson, coal-fired power companies, and the fishing industry could not hold back its publication indefinitely, thanks to nongovernment organizations such as the Sierra Club, NRDC, and others who were watching out for us. But even with this report, the FDA did not have to listen, comply, or do anything differently, since commercial fish fall in its jurisdiction, seemingly out of reach of the EPA report. Meanwhile, the coal-fired power plant companies would continue their deal making with our elected officials, in order to avoid the cost of reducing their pollution.

CHAPTER 17

Strategic Errors and Redundant Tactics

F ROM THE 1970s ON, polluting industries and the larger predatory fish industry have certainly been under siege, but so far they have been quite successful at defending their positions. Controlling pollution takes money to bring existing sources of mercury emissions into compliance. Admitting that the mercury content of fish comes primarily from such pollution and that a number of people who were exposed to it in quantity are adversely affected would be a heavy blow to all involved. The fishing industry and its lobbying groups are major believers that no person in the United States has ever had mercury poisoning from consuming oceangoing fish. At best, they will recognize only the "overt" symptomatology profile of mercury poisoning with its extreme effects, typically ignoring what's been called lesser Minamata, subjective methylmercury poisoning, or nonspecific symptoms of mercury poisoning. I prefer to call it simply fish fog. But whatever the name, the syndrome is the same. It exists and causes health problems for those who have it until they stop overexposing themselves. Unfortunately, no one knows at what point the lesser symptoms begin to cause permanent damage.

The arguments industry has used to forestall stringent regulations include these: It is legal to pollute; it is too expensive to reduce emissions; our emissions are not the cause of the pollution; someone else is the cause of the mercury discharge; if we reduce our emissions it won't matter because China is now the main offender; mercury is natural in the environment; our pollution is not enough to cause harm to humans; people do not eat enough fish for mercury to be a problem; and, best yet, a new directive states that mercury causes no harm, so it must not.

The real question in such matters for us, the public, is, who can we trust? The polluters? Or do we trust the government agencies in charge of regulating them? How about the people who are suing the industry? Let's not forget the scientists who may or may not have conducted an adequate study and the physicians who did not know there was mercury in fish in the first place.

When the Dow Chemical Company polluted the St. Clair River in Ontario, the company claimed that its mercury emissions were within Canada's legal guidelines. In other words, the company did no wrong. In the 1970s the State of Ohio and the Province of Ontario independently began proceedings to sue Dow Chemical of Sarnia and the parent company in Midland, Michigan, for the mercury pollution of Lake Erie and Lake St. Clair. The only compensation I've been able to find noted was in a Canadian press report indicating that in 1979 Dow paid $250,000 in an out-of-court settlement that Ontario then divided among the "affected" fishermen. (I took this to mean economically affected.) Canada has since set up multiple programs to compensate people who suffered adverse health effects caused by mercury pollution, but court battles are continuing today. Dow eventually shut down and dismantled the original Sarnia plant, then built a new one equipped with technology that can achieve zero mercury emissions.[1]

The official ban on commercial fishing in Canada's Ontario and Manitoba provinces lasted about nine years, from 1970 to 1978, until the fish in the polluted lakes and streams allegedly carried less than 0.5 mcg/g of mercury. Noncommercial fishing continued in this period, despite the mercury levels. In the United States, the fact that a number of researchers, who were funded in part by the fishing industry, interpreted the initial data from the Iraqi methylmercury seed grain poisoning to mean that adults were not affected by mercury until their blood levels were over 500 mcg/l, and that the children would have only "very very minimal effects," defined by Dr. Marsh in the case that rolled back the FDA's mercury guideline as retardation, seizures, slow to walk and talk, short stature, and small head,[2] when the mother had a blood mercury beginning at 400 mcg/l apparently saved the industry from further regulation. Industry "experts," using museum specimens, also delivered opinions on the "naturalness" of methylmercury in fish and gave the opinion without scientific evidence that selenium in fish helped protect against the effects of methylmercury, as we've seen. Those tactics worked·in the 1970s and on into the first years of the twenty-first century quite well. Are they still working?

At the end of 2000, mercury was added to the list of toxicants covered under the Clean Air Act as Bill Clinton was near the end of his term as president. President George W. Bush would then have to weigh economic interests on one side and public health on the other, with members of Congress pushing and pulling on both sides. It would be his responsibility to find a way to reduce mercury emissions from coal-fired power plants and other sources. Those who donated to his campaign seemed quite alert to this fact. If one looks at the recipients of money from the electric utilities in 2004, George Bush was number one, with $946,368; he was also the number one recipient of money from the coal mining industry, at $277,409.[3]

To come to a decision about mercury policy, the government had to assess not only the extent of emissions, but also the extent of public exposure to mercury and its dangers. The Centers for Disease Control has been evaluating public exposure to mercury among Americans every two years as part of a large-scale survey and blood sampling known as the National Health and Nutrition Examination Survey (NHANES). Some of these reports had been published in the CDC's *Morbidity and Mortality Weekly Report*, which physicians read. In the NHANES mercury report of November 2004, the CDC was pleased to say that the percentage of people in the U.S. population with more than 5.8 mcg/l of mercury in their blood was only 5.66. This was lower than in the NHANES report of 2001, when 8.0% of those surveyed had mercury blood levels that high. The CDC's 2001 report confirmed the Mahaffey and Keating risk estimate of significant mercury exposure of 7 percent to 10 percent, which, as you may recall, the Office of Management and Budget had reduced to 1 percent to 3 percent. As of 2008, the CDC has been unable to confirm the 1 to 3 percent risk level predicted by the OMB of 1995.[4]

The energy industry cheered the 2004 NHANES results, which it said indicated that the industry's efforts were yielding an improvement in the mercury levels of the American population. Some said there was no need for any regulation, as the current reductions were adequate. Under Bush's administration, the EPA proposed two regulatory alternatives to control emissions from coal- and oil-fired power plants. The first was to do as the EPA had planned in 2000: try to reduce mercury emissions as much as could be achieved using the best technology. The second was to implement a cap-and-trade system, which allows a company that owns both old polluting and newer, cleaner plants, for example, to get overall credit for pollution reduction, as the older polluting plants would be able to buy pollution credits from their less polluting counterparts. In March of 2005, the EPA chose the second and, in the process, removed mercury from the list of toxicants covered under the Clean Air Act.[5]

One objection often raised to the cap-and-trade provision can be simply expressed as a hypothetical question: Can you live in New Jersey with the polluting plants and breathe the air in Oregon that has fewer polluting plants? New Jersey did not think so, and together with many other states in the union, took the EPA to court. Members of the industry would now need to fight hard to keep mercury out from under the Clean Air Act, to gain more time to find new technologies that would lend us clean air, and phase out the old plants by death from natural causes.

NHANES was the study that the energy commission and industry lobbyists and others had relied on to help them influence policy. Although this survey was supposed to be representative of the U.S. population, it was not designed to look into subpopulations at risk, such as that of my patients. After all, they were deemed "unordinary." Regardless, it should at least be representative of the major various ethnic groups in the United States. I read with interest the CDC report in November 2004 that identified the percentages of racial and ethnic groups and their respective average mercury levels. Among the 5.66 percent of people in the NHANES mercury study population of 3,637 individuals that had blood mercury levels over 5.8 mcg/l, the report identified non-Hispanic black, non-Hispanic white, and Mexican American. When I added up the figures, I discovered that there were

360 individuals not identified in the tables whose data was used for the final analysis.[6]

Although NHANES data was selectively released to the public and was available on the Internet for research use, you had to have the right statistical program to download it properly and the knowledge of how to run the statistical program. Serendipitously, through the Internet I met Professor German Hernandez, MD, when he e-mailed a mercury question to me. He had just published a scientific paper using NHANES data and happened to have what I needed on his laptop. Together with Professor Ann O'Hare, MD, we began looking at the actual raw data. The two "other" categories of NHANES subjects not identified were what the NHANES raw data set referred to as "Other Hispanic" and "Other." The "Other" group consisted of individuals who self-identified as Asians, Pacific Islanders, Native Americans, and multiracial people. After putting the data through the proper statistical calculations, we discovered that in that category, 16.59 percent were over the 5.8 mcg/l level of mercury in the blood.[7]

It was not surprising to anyone that this "Other" group as a whole had a higher prevalence of elevated mercury levels, as many among them were known to consume fish regularly in their diet. Why this disparity was not revealed to the medical community and the group at risk was a curious question that the CDC has failed to answer. For California, Alaska, Washington, Oregon, and Hawaii, this group was especially important. In the 2000 United States Census, 4.1 million people identified themselves as Native American or Alaskan Native and 12.5 million as Asian or Pacific Islander, with 51 percent residing in the West.

Before my NHANES article stating that Asians, Pacific Islanders, and Native Americans were more commonly found to have elevated mercury levels than other racial and ethnic groups was published, the U.S. Tuna Foundation boasted that a "comprehensive" report released January 1, 2005, by Resources Committee chairman Richard Pombo (R-CA) and Energy and Mineral Resources Subcommittee chairman Richard Gibbons (R-NV) of the U.S. House of Representatives affirmed that the "health benefits of consuming seafood far outweigh any risk due to the trace amounts of mercury in some fish." They also declared that the government NHANES survey did not show anyone at risk.[8]

The key spin words here were "trace" and "some." Were they identifying the high-mercury fish as having trace mercury? Or were they referring to the low-mercury fish, what I as a clinician would refer to as trace-mercury fish, such as sardines? It was those unidentified "some" fish that seemed to be confusing us all as well. When it comes to humans and exposures, all things are relative. What defined "trace" when it comes to mercury was yet to be determined. Ardent fish consumers continued to be ignored. The raw data of NHANES included pregnant women with mercury levels greater than 10 mcg/l in their blood. Unfortunately, these people, and their mercury levels, got statistically cancelled out within the framework of the overall statistical conclusions. It does not mean they do not exist, though.

In dismissing claims of mercury's harm from eating fish, Gibbons and Pombo remarked, "It is impossible to craft and implement good public policy in a climate of fear."[9] I agree fully with that statement, but I have the opposite approach. Leaving people in the dark only breeds more fear. Educating them and making them aware of a situation will allow them to make an educated decision. None of my patients were ever "scared." Perhaps angry, let down, sad, or betrayed, but this resulted in their quickly becoming educated. Some patients were guided by their own experiences at sea. I once asked two retired navy officers independent of one another if they ate fish. They both expressed the same concern and stated, "I don't eat fish." They then remarked in an almost identical way that they knew what they had thrown over-board, but God only knew what the other guys threw over. Now that was scary.

Pombo and Gibbons declared in their report that China was to blame for a large portion of the current mercury emissions, though acknowledging the existence of 1,100 coal-fired power plants in the United States that used 1.004 billion tons of coal in 2003 and provided 52 percent of the nation's electricity. He said that those U.S. power plants emitted less than 1 percent of the annual world total. According to the *Mercury Study Report*, however, 33 percent of the mercury emissions in the United States had been coming from coal-fired power plants and were the single largest emission source. In 2007, a report from the BioDiversity Research Institute concluded, "Local mercury emissions are linked to elevated local deposition and high mercury in biota." Coal-fired power plants were implicated as being the major contributor to regional "hot spots" for mercury contamination.[10]

Pombo and Gibbons also included in their report a Department of Energy quote to the effect that "there was no commercially available technology that could consistently and cost-effectively capture mercury from coal-based power plants."[11] If the emissions of toxic fumes of many types, including mercury, can be reduced in factories, cars, waste incinerators, crematoria, and the like, they could be reduced in coal-fired power plants, as well. Using coal that emits lower amounts of mercury would also help. Perhaps the problem was that the power companies did not want to regulate the coal mines and their own generating plants, the fishing industry did not want to regulate the power companies, the FDA did not want to regulate the fishing industry, and the restaurants and grocery stores did not want to regulate the customer's consumption. It is an unwritten rule in business that one industry not call for the regulation of another, as this may implicate the identified industry in wrongdoing, or cause an increase in cost, or come back to haunt the complaining industry leaders. Regardless of who was at fault for the extent of mercury in fish, perhaps something will be figured out as many more people switch to nonfish sources of omega-3 fatty acids and use supplements instead of eating fish high on the food chain to meet the American Heart Association's recommendations for a healthy diet.

Some of the influential medical establishments, too, were having difficulty separating their science from their bank accounts. The American Heart Association placed itself in an ethical bind in 1990 when it tried to institute a food endorsement program. Opposition from the FDA and some food groups brought a halt to the initial program, but five years later, the AHA instituted its "Heart Healthy" label endorsement program. The AHA has been an advisory source for the public for many years, and its mission is to reduce disability and death from cardiovascular disease and stroke. However, the endorsed companies pay the AHA to place the "Heart Healthy" label on their products. StarKist was the first canned tuna product to be endorsed by the heart association. The company paid extra for exclusivity and even in 2008 remained the only readily visible canned fish product in the grocery store that carried this special endorsement from the AHA. No fresh fish was listed as being endorsed by the program. The only frozen fish endorsed by AHA as of June 2008 were frozen Arctic Surf clams, Hawaiian Pacific ahi, Orange Roughy fillets, and Chesapeake Bay Gourmet Crab Cakes.[12]

Many food companies have given millions of dollars to the American Heart Association either directly or indirectly through fund-raisers. The AHA has been publishing papers in its journals not only about the good health effects of omega-3 fatty acids, but also showing that methylmercury may negate the good effects of omega-3 fatty acids and could increase heart attacks and risk of stroke. Curiously, level of methylmercury content has not been a part of the criteria used to grant use of the "Heart Healthy" label.

Although the AHA has come a long way in developing Web sites that address mercury and omega-3 fatty acid content, it is behind on its mercury consumption tables, as they allow a mercury consumption of 30 mcg/day. This dose is what was considered safe by the WHO in 1977, and would result in a blood mercury level of about 23 mcg/l in a 132-pound person. This level exceeds what is considered safe for cardiovascular health in recent scientific papers. Lynda Knobeloch from the Wisconsin State Department of Health and Family Services and I wrote a polite letter to the CEO of the American Heart Association in 2005 pointing out this discrepancy. We never received a reply.[13]

With all the political interpretations of scientific reports and scientists' political interpretations of what their own data meant, it was no wonder that most everyone has been confused about mercury issues. This confusion and alleged decline in the public's purchase of some species of large predatory fish led the National Oceanic and Atmospheric Administration to ask the Institute of Medicine of the National Academy of Sciences to review the mercury and health literature and give an advisory. NAS released its report in October 2006. It triggered a hurricane of confusing reports in the media. This confusion was mainly because the fish industry fed the media their headline, to the effect that the benefits of fish outweighed the risk of contaminants. What some of the media reports did not tell you was the other half of the NAS's conclusions that two 3-ounce servings of a variety of fish per week was the point up to which the benefits outweighed the risk. The NAS statement that may have been most perplexing to the consumer was, "The scientific evidence about benefits and risk, however, is diverse, somewhat incomplete, and uncertain. Because of this uncertainty, the committee determined that no easy equation adequately expresses the complexity of the benefit and risk trade-offs involved in making seafood choices."[14]

In other words, eat at your own risk, because we give up.

The NAS panel, therefore, simply reiterated the FDA's advisory for children and pregnant women. It said women who were pregnant, might become pregnant, or were breast-feeding could reasonably consume two 3-ounce (cooked) servings but could safely consume 12 ounces per week. The differences between "reasonably" and "safely" were not defined.

The NAS advice that people could consume up to 6 ounces of white albacore tuna per week was heavily criticized by many experts, as consuming this much albacore would exceed the EPA's reference dose for many women and children. Also, there were many other fish that experts agreed should be on the do-not-eat list for these sensitive groups. The advice I give to my patients for commercial fish is don't eat a fish that is larger than your plate, with the exception of wild salmon. For noncommercial fish, fish eaters need to check the advisory for where the fish was obtained to determine consumption information.

The good thing was that the NAS addressed the rest of the population, as well as those at cardiovascular risk, which was a welcome change to the "let's kinda warn 'em" approach of the FDA. For healthy adolescents and adult males and females, the report stated that one can reduce risk of future cardiovascular disease by consuming seafood regularly. The NAS then advised that those who consume more than two servings per week should ensure that they select a variety of seafood to reduce the risk for exposure to contaminants from a single source. Those adults at risk for coronary heart disease, it said, "may" reduce their risk for cardiovascular disease by consuming seafood regularly, "although supporting evidence is limited."[15] Keep in mind, if one chose the low-mercury-content fish in their variety, one would avoid the mercury issue altogether.

Concurrently, a paper by Dariush Mozaffarian and Eric Rimm released in the *Journal of the American Medical Association* (JAMA) also confused many media commentators and others. It covered the risk and benefits of consuming fish and took into consideration mercury and PCBs, cardiovascular risk, and cancer risk (from PCBs). Part of the problem was that both the Mozaffarian and Rimm paper and the NAS reports were released to the media and some special interest groups before being made available to the general public. This left a behind-the-scenes scramble to digest the reports prior to public release so that the rebuttals and supportive comments could be made on the day of their official release. Contributing to this confusion were the authors' edited-down conclusions in the JAMA paper, the industry spin tactics, and the lack of understanding among some journalists of what the reports actually said.

In the JAMA abstract, the conclusion stated, "For major outcomes among adults, based on both the strength of the evidence and the potential magnitudes of effect, the benefits of fish intake exceed the potential risk. For women of childbearing age, benefits of modest fish intake, excepting a few selected species, also outweigh risks."[16]

The key phrase here was "modest fish intake." In the body of the paper that was defined as one 6-ounce or two 3-ounce servings of fish per week.

The JAMA authors stated that selenium "may" reduce tissue accumulation of mercury in fish and humans and said therefore additional investigation was warranted. They referenced a paper that reported a reduction, by selenium, in mercury excretion in the hair of twenty-three human subjects. They noted that the literature on selenium and mercury is still contradictory and that any protective effect of selenium has not been proven.[17]

The key points Mozaffarian and Rimm and the academy made were that the effects of low-level methylmercury exposure in adults have not been established, and that mercury may modestly reduce the cardiovascular benefits of fish intake; therefore, the authors recommended that consumers choose fish with higher omega-3 fatty acid content and lower mercury levels.[18] The basic message given by much of the media and the industry, though, was that the benefits outweighed the risk, end of story. This sent a dangerous message to high-end consumers to eat as much as they wanted. For those who cannot get fish past their lips, two 3-ounce servings seem like mountains—for my high-end consumers, 3 ounces is something you put on a cracker.

For the poor, the albacore tuna issue was being heavily fought behind the scenes. Many individuals and environmental groups tried to get albacore tuna removed from the federally funded Women Infants Children program because of its mercury content. Public health officials from Hawaii had also requested that their WIC people be allowed other canned fish or meat products than albacore. This request by Hawaii was granted seemingly with ease.

The federally funded WIC was a program that gave vouchers for the purchase of select food items—including 24 ounces of albacore tuna per month—to pregnant or nursing mothers. Participants had no other nondairy protein options. Finally, quietly, after much debate and deliberation, on August 7, 2006, the *Federal Register* announced a proposed rule that stated, "For ease of administration by State agencies, to accommodate participant preferences, and to minimize intake of mercury, this proposed rule would authorize the following varieties of canned fish—light tuna, salmon, and sardines." The U.S. Department of Agriculture also proposed to raise the amount of canned fish allowed to 30 ounces per month. Albacore, it appeared, was no longer allowed to be purchased with the federal government voucher.[19]

This expansion of the WIC canned protein allowance was certainly a step in the right direction. What did the Tuna Foundation make of this? Its astonishing headline of an August 2006 press release was

"Science Shows WIC Moms and Children Will Reap Health Benefits from More Canned Tuna." In the first line of her statement, the president of the foundation wrote, "The proposed new food list for the women, infants and children (WIC) nutrition program, published today in the Federal Register, takes an important step toward improving the health of low-income women and children it serves by increasing allowances for women for canned tuna, a highly nutritious, heart-healthy fish."[20]

So now that the federal government had removed albacore from WIC because of its mercury content, one would think the FDA would be prompted to reexamine other of its mercury and fish advisories. But there's no clear move so far in that direction. For the FDA, the WIC program change wasn't a precedent. WIC, it turns out, is run by the U.S. Department of Agriculture, and not the FDA.

If regulation of mercury in commercial fish is still an open issue, so, too, is control of mercury at one of its prime sources, coal-fired power companies. The EPA had delisted mercury under the Clean Air Act, but was this justified? The United States Court of Appeals decided in February of 2008 that the EPA had no authority to delist mercury from the Clean Air Act without taking the steps required under the act. Therefore, a more stringent control of mercury pollution from this source could be coming soon. Just don't hold your breath in anticipation.[21]

CHAPTER 18

The Canning of Proposition 65 Mercury Warnings

FOR THIRTY-SEVEN YEARS, ever since the first mercury scare, the tuna and swordfish industries have been the most vociferous when it comes to methylmercury in fish. The U.S. Tuna Foundation, especially, has continually defended its position that mercury is natural and causes no harm, that no person eats enough fish for the mercury ingested to cause harm, and that there has never been a case of mercury toxicity from consuming oceangoing fish in the United States.

By 1986, California's citizens had heard enough discussion of scientific controversies and arguments over pollution regulation and the need to guard the public against toxic exposures of all sorts to want to see some action. At that time, opinion polls indicated that danger posed by toxic waste was the number one fear among Californians. Out of this concern, the state referendum called Proposition 65 was born and was passed by the voters in 1986 by a significant margin. Proposition 65 prohibits the knowing and intentional exposure of an individual to a chemical known to the State of California to cause cancer or reproductive harm without first giving clear and reasonable warning to such individual.

Methylmercury, under Prop 65, was a candidate for such a warning. With more information about the harmful effects of methylmercury coming from the Faroes study, the *Mercury Study Report*, and my high-end consumer survey, nongovernment watchdog groups began pressing the California attorney general to uphold the statute and post warnings where mercury-laden fish, including canned tuna, was sold. Court battles ensued, which resulted in requiring methylmercury-in-fish warnings for California restaurants and grocery stores to be posted, beginning in February 2003. But, as the manufacturers of canned tuna well knew, there are exceptions to every rule. They did not want the warnings on or near their cans and did not feel a warning for their product was necessary under the statute.

Some years earlier, in 1998, the attorney general (AG) of California, Bill Lockyer, took on the task of determining whether canned tuna needed a Prop 65 warning for its methylmercury content. A meeting took place in March with the AG; a representative of the Office of Environmental Health Hazard Assessment; and David Burney, executive director of the San Diego–based U.S. Tuna Foundation, which represented California's tuna industry.

At the meeting, it was mentioned that new results of the Seychelles mercury study would be coming out. Even though the paper was not to be published for several more months, Burney told the attorney general's office that Thomas Clarkson of the University of Rochester was willing to come to California to discuss the results. The follow-up meeting took place that May. Clarkson was not on the officially recorded guest list for the May meeting, nor did he officially sign in, but Burney said the tuna industry brought him along.[1]

Clarkson, according to Burney's testimony during the *People of California vs Tri-Union Seafoods et al.* court proceedings[2] in 2006, told the attorney general that the Seychelles study had not found an adverse effect from consumption of mercury-laden fish and that the Seychelles population's mercury levels were comparable to what would be expected in the U.S. population. Clarkson differentiated between the Seychelles study that was basically conducted on a fish-consuming population, and the Faroes study, whose population also consumed large amounts of whale meat and whale blubber. He apparently also mentioned that the Faroes Islands had the highest percentage of PCBs ever recorded in a mammal (whales) and that this was a "confounder" that had to be resolved. Because of the amount of naturally occurring methylmercury in the seas, Burney claimed, Prop 65 was not a requirement for canned fish. The tuna industry would later say that because the attorney general's office took no further action on this matter after the 1998 meetings, the industry believed it was in compliance with Prop 65 and no warning label was needed.[3]

All went well for the industry until nongovernment watchdog groups began their own testing of canned tuna and found it to contain more mercury than the amount claimed in 1998 that had precluded the industry from Prop 65 warnings. In 2001, one of these groups, Public Media Center (PMC), filed private notices of violation against the tuna canners. The Sea Turtle Restoration Project followed with another notice of violation in 2002. My high-end consumer survey, which was coincidental to all of this, was first presented on October 1, 2002.

It is understandable to me now why reporting on mercury poisoning in my patients who consumed a lot of commercial fish caused such a stir at the time. Although I did not fully address symptoms in the paper, I suspected that the symptoms of many of my patients could be traced to methylmercury, and a court could have recognized my observations as a witness for those patients. I would not have had to prove anything, just tell the court what my observations were and show that my patients' symptoms were consistent with mercury exposure, as reported in the literature—of which was so aggressively suppressed in the past in Japan, Canada, Iraq, and elsewhere. The industry knew people had come forward long before my patients did to voice their experience with this syndrome that occurs at the lower mercury exposure levels. The industry was able to hold back the tide in the 1970s, but now that people could get their blood tested so easily and accurately, they could come forward in increasing numbers and make it more difficult for industry to deny their claims.

Industry claimed that the recent notice of violations by PMC and others were filed without new evidence, essentially ignoring the new testing of people who consumed its product. Another court intervention, industry felt, was not necessary.[4] The new information led the attorney general to take over the suit filed by the NGOs against the tuna canners. After all, my study showed that pregnant women, women of childbearing age, and children were consuming large predator fish, including canned tuna, and had elevated mercury levels because of it. The problem, though, was that the statute provided protection only for those who had "reasonable" or "average" consumption patterns.

You know, "ordinary." High-end consumers had not been considered ordinary; therefore, they were essentially on their own.[5]

Because an out-of-court agreement could not be reached on the labeling of canned tuna, in January of 2003 the people of the State of California and Attorney General Bill Lockyer faced Tri-Union Seafoods LLC, Del Monte Corporation, Bumble Bee Seafoods LLC, et al., in the superior court of the state of California, city and county of San Francisco, with Judge Robert Dondero presiding. I awaited the judge's decision with tremendous interest; by this day and time, there surely was enough scientific literature about mercury to allow for a clear and reasonable warning in regard to mercury and canned tuna.

I was quite confused, though, when I read the proposed ruling documents by the plaintiffs and then read the decision of April 17, 2006. Judge Dondero's decision was a cut-and-paste and mostly word-for-word montage of the industry's proposed rulings. He did not even remove the industry's document tracking number that was evident on "his" decision document. Here is what transpired, and it can serve as another lesson in how the laws, courts, and some government agencies have been protecting us.[6]

First of all, the tuna industry asked the FDA to intervene before the trial began and requested a letter to the California attorney general stating that the FDA's federal advisory preempted the state's Proposition 65 warning. In his decision, Dondero stated, "FDA has studied carefully the issue of methylmercury in fish for more than twenty-five years and had developed substantial expertise in analyzing both the scientific and consumer education aspects of the issue." He went on to say, "The FDA's policy on warning labels on food has been a nuanced approach, where ingredient and nutrition information is disclosed, and warnings are required only under exceptional circumstances, such as when food has been adulterated or misbranded. It is FDA's position that warning over-exposure could lead consumers to ignore all warnings, which could create an even greater public health problem."[7]

Judge Dondero even quoted a fishing industry expert witness, a Dr. Louis Sullivan, who claimed that "a label statement that reaches the general public can have unintended adverse public health consequences, such as reduced consumption." He went on: "FDA's policy approach in the FDA/EPA advisory specifically avoids warning all consumers in favor of a more comprehensive targeted approach."[8]

As a physician who continued to see the people who were victims of this type of "targeted" or "nuanced" approach, who actually did need to reduce their consumption, it all seemed like frustrating gibberish. It's hard to imagine the far worse heartache experienced by the sufferers of mercury poisonings in Canada and Japan who were very seriously affected yet had to sit through the flailing about of official after official during their years of abuse.

Proposition 65 only covered reproductive toxicity or harm and cancer. So much of the scientific literature got left on the shelf when it came to mercury policy making. Methylmercury had not been associated with cancer; therefore, the statute in regard to methylmercury would only apply to women having babies and to infants. Men and non-reproductive women were not the target population. Not because they could not be harmed, but because the statute just did not recognize them. For a physician, this disparity was unacceptable, as it meant that cardiovascular disease, autoimmune disease, neuropsychiatric effects, subjective complaints, and male infertility associated with methylmercury would not be in play in the trial. Evidence that methylmercury had been shown to adversely affect sperm production and had been correlated with reduced fertility in men in several studies, was not argued before the court, that I could find.[9] Aren't men's sperm part of the reproductive system?

In Dondero's interpretation, "The objective of the 2004 FDA/EPA advisory was to inform the target population of women who may become pregnant, pregnant women, nursing mothers, and parents of young children how to get the positive health benefits from eating fish and shellfish, while minimizing their exposure to methylmercury."[10]

The judge claimed that the FDA had made efforts to inform the targeted audience through a comprehensive education campaign that included publication of a consumer-oriented magazine, development of videos, and dissemination of information through its offices of consumer affairs and public affairs. He also declared that the FDA sent information to physicians, other health professionals, and health care associations to distribute through their offices.[11]

Interesting. As a practicing California physician, I certainly had not received any such materials at my office, and I had yet to find a colleague who had.

A critical provision of the Prop 65 statute indicated that if a person could show that exposure to the given chemical would have no observable effect at a dose that was one thousand times less than what was known to have an adverse effect or cause harm, a warning was not required. This exposure was referred to as the maximum allowable dose level (MADL).

According to the fishing companies' conclusions, of which Judge Dondero approved, a no-observable-effect level (NOEL) had to be obtained in order to derive a maximum allowable dose level. Dondero essentially accepted the industry's notion that the Iraqi study, ostensibly to demonstrate that its estimated no-observable-effect level was so low that it would be scientifically difficult to defend. This statement in the judge's decision seemed illogical and clearly represented an industry plea. In the 1977 Anderson trial, fishing industry expert witnesses used preliminary data from Iraq to convince the judge that one could consume 300 mcg of mercury per day without harm. But because subsequent papers from Iraq showed that much lower mercury levels were associated with effects, we're led to believe that the data should no longer be used at a trial. This argument was of course nonsensical, but evidently convincing to the court.

Judge Dondero approvingly referenced the testimony of F. Jay Murray, the defense team's expert toxicologist. Murray said he had reviewed more than thirty epidemiological and animal studies to determine the most appropriate study on which to base an MADL for methylmercury. A rat study of 1980 conducted by M. Bornhausen of Germany represented the "best quality" and yielded the lowest no-observable-effect level, according to Murray. In this study, sixteen pregnant rats were given varying doses of methylmercury on four different days during their pregnancy. The subsequent eighty pups were then put through a series of tests, including training to press levers to obtain food. A no-observable-effect point of 5 mcg/kg of body weight per day was determined.[12]

I read that study. To rely on sixteen rats and their eighty pups pushing levers to tell us how much mercury was safe for humans to consume without damage was utterly pathetic. At Bornhausen's no-observable-effect level, a 132-pound person could consume 300 mcg a day (and presumably still be able to learn to pull a lever). Doesn't that number seem familiar? Oh, I get it. *This* is today's magic number. That 132-pound person would have an estimated 225mcg/l blood mercury level with this amount. Neither the Iraqi data nor any of the human studies, including the Seychelles study, support this amount of exposure as being safe any longer. Therefore, they had to look for a study that did. Rats!

Further dividing this 300 mcg/day value by 1,000 gave a maximum allowable daily dose of 0.3 mcg/day. The tuna industry knew that this was the number it needed to keep the warnings off tuna. This would be more or less equivalent to consuming five cans of albacore per day.

What about the Faroes study? Judge Dondero quoted industry expert complaints that the Faroes study did not meet the requirements of Prop 65 because it failed to have both an exposed and a reference group, because the exposure was not limited to the prenatal period, and because PCB and DDT levels in the whales were confounding factors. As you may recall, the University of Rochester's Seychelles group calculated that fetal effects on humans occurred at a blood level of about 80 mcg/l. It seems the fishing industry had no use for the Rochester group's study, either.

Deborah Rice testified on behalf of the attorney general. Although a graduate from the University of Rochester, she is a vigorous critic of industry tactics and disagreed with just about everything the industry experts had opined at the trial. Her major points were that adverse effects in infants and children were seen at exposures less than what the industry proposed; that one large dose could affect the fetus; that other animals were different from humans and the no-observable-effect level needed to be adjusted, as rats tolerate much more mercury than humans; and that for Prop 65 the benchmark dose of the Faroes was an adequate measure of the maximum allowable dose level. Therefore, blood mercury of 58 mcg/l would be where fetal effects were seen.

For a final blast to confidence in the effectiveness of the "new math" in the tuna trial, consider two greatly debated major points that would decide how to make the final calculations. First, the industry witnesses said there was no proof that one dose of methylmercury above the maximum allowable dose determined would cause harm; therefore, the mercury levels in the cans of tuna should be averaged and the range of mercury levels should not be used. (Canned tuna mercury levels vary widely by can and therefore have a range of levels.) Then they argued that, according to their consumption survey, the average pregnant woman consumed only 64.4 g of tuna on average every sixty days; therefore, the consumption rate should be averaged over two months. Next, of course, were arguments at the trial about what "average" meant.[13]

Murray proceeded with all his calculations to come up with the perfect number, just as Crispin-Smith had in the 1977 Anderson trial. He averaged everything he could, including the lower-mercury chunk light average with the higher-mercury albacore average, then adding the two and averaging that. Without all the averages of averages, the labels would be on the cans, despite the sixteen rat mothers and their eighty pups. Using the industry's methods for albacore alone would have meant that the albacore would require a label and the chunk light would not. When it comes to our health, this kind of averaging is ridiculous, of course. Regardless, Judge Dondero ruled that the industry case contained adequate proof that no labels need be present on any can of tuna.

The last point on which the industry had needed to convince the judge was that the methylmercury in canned tuna was natural. According to Dondero, human consumption of a food was not an "exposure" to a listed chemical for the purposes of Prop 65 if it was "naturally occurring"; a natural constituent of a food; or absorbed or accumulated from an environment where it was naturally present and where the food was raised, grown, or obtained. A chemical was naturally occurring only to the extent that it did not result from any known human activity.

In one part of the trial, industry and subsequently Judge Dondero claimed that methylmercury in fish was 100 percent natural. According to them, elemental mercury was the main form of mercury that was emitted from power plants into the atmosphere, elemental mercury was not the type of mercury that existed in "trace amounts" in fish, and methylmercury was not emitted from power plants. This was like saying flour was not responsible for bread. The power plants emit mercury into the air, it falls to the ground or sea, bacteria there convert it to methylmercury, and it then enters the food chain. If there weren't so much mercury in the air, there might not be as much methylmercury in the fish.

The key witness industry called to demonstrate that methylmercury was natural was François Morel from Princeton University. He had been conducting some experiments in water bodies to discern where and how mercury gets converted to methylmercury. He had concluded that in the ocean, this conversion takes place in a layer that is not accessible to human pollution, and that somehow hydrothermal vents in the deep sea were the real source of methylmercury in fish. He thought at least 95 percent of the methylmercury in fish was naturally occurring, while the state's witness, William Fitzgerald, thought that 50 to 75 percent of ocean methylmercury was naturally occurring. The judge somehow concluded from this that it was "indisputable that methylmercury was not deposited in the ocean as a result of industrial pollution."[14]

Dr. Morel also wrote a paper comparing the mercury levels in museum specimens to those of fresh fish and used this at trial to say the levels have not changed over time. This paper was partially funded by the U.S. Tuna Foundation.[15]

After the twenty-four-day trial, hundreds of pages of post-trial discussion, and the judge's decision, the attorney general struck back. In his letter of objection to the proceedings, Lockyer said that he felt the court had signed off on the defendant's one-sided version of the law and the facts without addressing the state's arguments and objections. The result was a ruling that was "legally and factually unsupportable, and that incorporates defendants' distortions, misinterpretations, and biases."[16]

Lockyer noted several times that the court's decision adopted every proposed finding submitted by the defendants nearly verbatim, even when the findings were flatly contradicted by the law and the record. Among the "indefensible errors" noted were the following:

- That the Court would reject the use of the best epidemiological studies, and the views of the leading scientific organizations in the world, including the United States EPA, establishing the toxicity of methylmercury.
- That the Court would find that even where a chemical was present in food as a result of industrial pollution, it was considered "naturally occurring," even though the applicable regulation expressly states to the contrary.
- That the Court would adopt the incorrect proposition that a pregnant woman's exposure to methylmercury could be averaged over a sixty day time period. This was because there was undisputable evidence from experimental data that a single exposure to methylmercury could cause developmental harm.
- That the Court would adopt the defendant's unsupportable assumption that a woman could ingest 300 mcg of methylmercury—the equivalent of eating what is in two swordfish steaks—on every day of her pregnancy, without causing harm to the fetus.

The AG noted that "there was not a reputable scientist or scientific body in the world today that would agree with Dr. Murray that 300 mcg/day was a 'no observable effect level' for methylmercury."[17]

The AG's expert witness Rice calculated a human maximum allowable dose level of 0.005 mcg/d; the AG stated that the court failed to consider relevant evidence concerning the proper way to calculate the maximum allowable dose level under Proposition 65, as the benchmark dose analysis was indeed permitted under the statute. He also made clear that PCBs in the Faroes were not found by the scientists to confound the methylmercury results nor invalidate them.

I asked Dr. Philippe Grandjean of the Faroes study whether he had ever been asked to be involved in any way in the issue of Prop 65 and methylmercury in tuna. After all, it was his study that was being stomped on at the play yard. He said he could not recall ever being asked to participate.[18]

The AG also discredited the studies using museum or comparison specimens because they were inadequate. He attacked Morel's testimony that methylmercury in tuna comes from the deep ocean by saying it was based entirely on hypothesis and theory and was not shared by any other scientist in the field.

It was well accepted that the tuna canners had not placed methylmercury into their product. It was not the tuna canners' fault that some people ate so much of it. Or was it? The fact that their cans said a serving size was two ounces and many people ate all six ounces, typically a can's contents, indicated that there were individuals who did not read labels. On the other hand, there continued to be a strong campaign by organizations such as the tuna industry, the American Heart Association, and the FDA to push fish health claims and to specifically include canned tuna in their recommendations.

Now, you might think the story would end there. But not with claims about mercury. A few months after the conclusion of the trial, a graduate student under Morel's supervision at Princeton University presented a poster entitled "Possible Biotic and Abiotic Sources of Methylmercury in the Ocean" at the Mercury 2006 conference in Madison, Wisconsin. Morel was scheduled to give a presentation at the conference, as well, but it was cancelled and changed to a poster presentation only at the request of the lead author. Morel was listed as the fourth author for the poster.[19]

In the project described, the researchers used DNA analysis to find out what types of bacteria were involved in the methylation of mercury in the ocean and at what depths methylation occurred. They discovered that it was facultative anaerobes (which can live in oxic and anoxic environments) such as *Vibrio* and *Aeromonas* that did the methylation and did so in the more oxic environment—that is, closer to the water surface, where the process could be reached by human pollution. The researchers also concluded that sulfate-reducing bacteria were not involved, as Morel had claimed, and that hydrothermal vents were not a significant source of methylmercury in the ocean, countering everything Morel had said in his testimony.[20] In other words, a member of his own research team disproved what Morel said in his influential testimony at the trial.

The AG went to the judge to request that the case be reopened and the poster entered as new evidence. Despite the evidence, Morel allegedly said he simply did not agree with the poster, and the judge subsequently denied the request to reopen the case.

For now, there is no system that adequately warns the public about how much methylmercury is in fish and what precautions people should take in California or elsewhere in the United States. The FDA's methylmercury Web page will be read only by those interested individuals who have Internet access. This certainly places at a disadvantage the poor, the computer illiterate, and those who do not know to go to the Internet to check the FDA advisories for whatever food they enjoy. So much for a "nuanced" approach. No mention of mercury—in a warning or in the list of ingredients—will appear on canned tuna for now. The California case's decision is on appeal, as of January 2008; however, the Proposition 65 methylmercury warnings for fish, that make more public the FDA advisory, at least continue to be posted for those who need or want them in restaurants and grocery stores in California—but not near the canned tuna.

CHAPTER 19

Diagnosis Mercury

WHEN I BEGAN INVESTIGATING my patients' elevated blood mercury, I sought to gain a clear understanding of how mercury affects one's health. When information was not at my fingertips, I wondered why. What began as an investigation to help me diagnose mercury-related symptoms in my patients grew into another diagnosis —that of a broken, misused, and abused regulatory system. The entire regulatory process needs an overhaul, along with the way we assess environmental factors in disease. The current system is still too susceptible to abuses from corporations that pay "scientists" to say whatever it is they want them to say, and to have undue influence over the writing of government reports and policy. The researchers who have the least amount of bias are often the ones not attached to any big money-gathering organizations and are therefore poorly funded to do careful and much-needed research on the effects of environmental toxicants. Some of our brightest researchers will continue to be recruited by the industry that has the finances to hire them; therefore, open books and peer review will be important factors to ensure that their science is sound.

In the global scheme, methylmercury, whether natural or added by humans, is in our fish. The distinction of natural versus adulterated has no bearing on how I address individuals at risk in my office. The argument of natural versus adulterated exists only because of how lawmakers and the food industry wrote the rules of labeling for disclosure to the consumer. It is a way to escape tighter regulation on unhealthful contaminants in food and allow the food industry to sell its products without much challenge to the contaminants' health effects.

As for coal-fired power plants and other industries that emit mercury, we at least need to enforce the present laws to keep mercury and other toxicants from further contaminating the environment. China is a long-recognized major contributor to the world's mercury pollution. The many smokestacks bellowing out mercury and other toxicants can affect the health of the people in that nation as well as their neighbors. Locally deposited mercury finds its way into the fish and other foods. China is a fish-loving nation, but so is the United States. We have coal-fired power plants that emit mercury, too, and they deposit their toxicants locally and broadly. For every 10 mcg/l elevation in blood mercury for a pregnant woman, there can be a drop in the intelligence quotient (IQ) of the child. A drop in intelligence of only five points over a population means fewer people in the very smart category and more who will need extra help in their lives, resulting not only in many lost personal opportunities but also in a strain on the society. Researchers have estimated the impact of lower IQ from power plant mercury emissions for the lifetime of the individual in regard to diminished economic productivity alone—for a cohort of exposed children in the United States, the loss was estimated to be about $8 billion annually (dollars in 2000).[1] While there have been gains in pollution abatement in the United States since the early 1970s, much is yet to be accomplished, and mercury remains a relatively neglected area.

In 1975, W. Eugene Smith wrote in the prologue to *Minamata* that when he was about to venture to Japan to investigate the Minamata disaster in the early 1970s, a scientist at a conference on mercury in Rochester approached to ask, "Why go there? It's finished in Minamata. What are you going to find to photograph?" Smith went on, "Not only did we find that 'it' was not finished, but we became convinced that 'it'—whether the poison is mercury, or asbestos, or food additives, or radiation, or something else—is closing more tightly upon us each day. Pollution growth is still running far ahead of any anti-pollution conscience."[2] The scientist who thought the Smiths did not need to go to Japan, according to Aileen Smith, was, ironically, Thomas Clarkson.[3]

In 2008, our regulatory system is still struggling to keep up with the polluters, and our health care team is still in the dark when it comes to environmental toxicants. As for mercury, recognizing the subjective symptoms from overexposure that precede "overt" toxicity is important to diagnose. Those who have the lesser symptoms—such as fatigue, headache, upset stomach, and the like—also have reduced productivity, as they incur more days off of work and are not as productive when they are at work. One of my patients in the mercury study went on temporary disability, while two others took early retirement. The patients who had side effects from their mercury exposure also incurred medical bills in the thousands of dollars in order to confirm the diagnosis. These expenses and distress could have been altogether avoided with better awareness on the part of the public and medical establishment and better attention from the FDA and other regulatory agencies. If we allow industry-funded researchers to define what constitutes toxicity, we run the risk of failing to properly diagnose and remedy the situation. As we've seen in one court case after another, there's been little focus on the serious harm that chronic mercury exposure may do, and the canneries and other interests have had a huge effect on what happens in these cases.

What, then, are the main concerns that are worrying researchers today about methylmercury?

As for children, because they are still growing brains and methylmercury interferes with a cell's ability to divide, the effects of methylmercury can be permanent. In-utero, chronic, low-end exposures show up later in school in the form of reduced performance on some tests of language, coordination, and intelligence. Adverse cardiac effects and other neurological and psychiatric effects are still being investigated.

As for childhood development in the face of methylmercury, more studies are certainly needed. Fortunately, a cohort study in the United States is now under way. In 1999–2002, 341 mother-child pairs in Massachusetts entered into a study to investigate the effects of mercury when the children were exposed in utero. The mother's red blood cells were tested for mercury in the second trimester. (0.0–9.0 mcg/l blood.) The authors, some of whom were consultants of the food industry, concluded that neurodevelopmental testing of the children at three years of age yielded the following observations: Modest mercury elevation was associated with lower childhood cognition at exposure levels substantially lower than in populations previously studied; no safe level for methylmercury was found in their study; and if mercury contamination was not present, the cognitive benefits of fish intake would be greater.[4]

As for what to do with such information, physicians and consumers need to be ever more diligent as to the types of fish and the quantity consumed, along with contaminant levels. In recent years, a number of health care workers and patients have called my office to ask my opinion as to what to do about an elevated mercury level found during a pregnancy. One woman, age thirty-eight, was twelve weeks pregnant with her first child when she discovered that her blood level was 48 mcg/l. The test was repeated and confirmed. The patient had seen on the news that there were high mercury levels in the fish that she had been consuming during pregnancy, so she asked her gynecologist for the test. When the result came in, her genetics counselor called to ask my opinion on the matter. Since there was no way to accurately predict the outcome for this mother's child, much soul searching transpired. She decided to go through with the pregnancy and delivered a healthy baby. It is too early to tell whether the child will have any adverse effects, but this mother decided to accept whatever was given to her regardless of any mercury effects that may become apparent in her child's future. Other women are now finding themselves in similar predicaments. Perhaps if the FDA practiced face-to-face clinical medicine with the public and realized the anguish of the people who are affected by the impact of mercury, they would stop hiding behind ghostly advisories and toothless policies.

When it comes to chronic methylmercury exposure with fish consumption in adults, research attention encompasses cardiovascular disease, nonspecific symptoms, adverse neuropsychiatric effects, infertility, and autoimmune effects.

The effects of mercury on the adult brain have been most commonly known in the hatters, but that was inorganic mercury. Now evidence is gathering that long-term methylmercury exposure can also lead to damage to the adult brain, including a diminished capacity to process information, reduced mental functioning, forgetfulness, insomnia, and abnormal eye movements. The threshold at which these effects will occur or become permanent is still being investigated, as we've seen; therefore, it would be wise not to chronically elevate your blood mercury level over 5 mcg/l.[5] Many of my fish-loving patients will get a blood mercury test as part of their physical exam to see if they are maintaining this. We also look at their diet as a whole and what they consumed in the week before the test, and then make adjustments as necessary.

Infertility induced by methylmercury exposure is a growing concern. Several studies indicate that chronic exposure to methylmercury can affect several aspects of semen: reduced concentration of sperm, lower percentage of morphologically normal sperm, lower percentage of mobile sperm, reduced velocity and less movement of sperm in general. These changes resulted in reduced fertility among men. Females with unexplained infertility also have sometimes been noted to have higher mercury levels.[6]

Perhaps the most difficult effect to sort out is the association of methylmercury with autoimmune disease. Autoimmune disease occurs when antibodies to one's own tissues and blood, called autoantibodies, are made. Humans are capable of making numerous autoantibodies, and new ones are discovered every year. Interestingly, multiple types of agents, including viruses and pollutants, can trigger their production in the human body. Not everyone can form these various autoantibodies, and genetic predisposition is a key factor in autoantibody production. That various forms of mercury can trigger production of autoantibodies in animals has been shown in a number of studies. Only recently has a similar mercury-induced process begun to be looked at in humans, and the threshold at which autoantibodies are triggered in genetically susceptible individuals currently remains unknown. People who themselves or whose family members have a history of autoimmune disease, such as lupus, thyroiditis, scleroderma, autoimmune kidney disease, or rheumatoid arthritis, should consume foods and omega-3 fatty acid supplements from sources that have little or no mercury contamination until further research can be conducted.[7]

When I looked at high-end fish consumers among my patient population, many of them not only had the symptoms that had been described throughout the literature, but also had diseases and conditions with which mercury had been correlated. Atherosclerosis, myocardial infarctions, strokes, autoantibodies, neuropsychiatric complaints, infertility, and nonspecific symptoms were all present in my study population and among subsequent patients coming to me for a mercury consultation. In medicine, we many times cannot prove cause and effect, but we can say that a symptom profile is consistent with a diagnosis. It is the in-the-trenches observations like these that could lead to larger studies so that the full spectrum of the effects of methylmercury on humans can be determined.

In the 1990s, Japanese researchers looked further into their "lesser Minamata" profile.[8] They identified subjective symptoms that could easily be missed or denied by patients with an economic interest in the outcome of the study or overstated by those wishing to win a lawsuit against the polluters. The researchers found statistically significant correlations between mercury consumption and symptoms studied as follows: muscle stiffness, dysesthesia (abnormal sensations, especially the sense of touch), hand tremor, dizziness, loss of pain sensation, muscle cramps, upper arm muscular atrophy, joint pain, back pain, leg tremor, ringing in the ears, muscular atrophy, chest pain, palpitations, fatigue, visual dimness, and staggering. Symptoms with statistical significance for men only were thirst and difficulty with urination. Those with statistical significance in women only were muscular weakness, urine incontinence, forgetfulness, and insomnia. The researchers concluded that chronic methylmercury poisoning shows a late onset of symptoms or an increase in symptoms after several years of exposure and has atypical and subclinical features unlike those of classic Minamata disease with its overt methylmercury symptoms. The problem with this study, though, was that the control population was still being exposed to methylmercury, so statistical significance for other symptoms could have been missed. My patient population had various of the above complaints and also hair loss, headache, trouble thinking and performing complex tasks, memory loss, insomnia, gastrointestinal upset, abdominal pain, metallic taste, and nausea. Those symptoms have also been reported in the literature in association with mercury exposure.[9]

My patients had symptoms that have been correlated with methylmercury exposure from fish consumption, and they had corresponding elevated mercury levels, along with chronic exposure to methylmercury that was consistent with the above study. Their diagnosis was therefore consistent with lesser Minamata. Regardless of how small the population or how unordinary, there are people in the United States who have lesser Minamata, mercury poisoning, or subjective methylmercury poisoning or fish fog, by consuming oceangoing fish. This syndrome continues to be suppressed by industry-funded researchers and the industries themselves—both the polluters and the fishing industry. It is still unclear to me what role the FDA is trying to play in this issue. Some people, like Bettye Russow, have overt methylmercury poisoning. Such sufferers have been here all the time, buried in the rat race and unrecognized.

Most of my patients appear to have recovered from their nonspecific symptoms after they stopped consuming the methylmercury and their blood levels went down to less than 5 mcg/l. Some took two to six months, while others took more than a year to recover, and a few claimed that their mental function was never the same. The ones who took longer to recover tended to be those who had autoantibodies such as antithyroglobulin, antimicrosomal, and antinucleolar antibodies. A curious finding was that five patients were diagnosed with autoimmune liver disease, which is not a common diagnosis. I had no autoimmune liver disease patients in the rest of my practice. The liver specialists and I have continued to follow those patients for the last seven years. More research needs to be done to see if there is a correlation between mercury and this disease, as the liver is a major organ in the body where mercury tends to accumulate-and mercury is known to stimulate autoantibodies.

Another important observation was that a few individuals who claimed no symptoms at all had blood mercury levels up to 29 mcg/l. Among the few children in my study, some have had persistent damage consistent with mercury exposure, such as trouble with learning and memory.

After I had the patients stop their mercury intake, or had them choose only low-mercury fish, the ones who had complained of muscle cramps had a curious experience. They would slowly get better after stopping the mercury consumption, then, when the mercury levels were approaching the point where they would be expected to be less than 2 mcg/l in blood, severe muscle cramps would occur for a day or two. The patients would feel better thereafter. Other colleagues have observed this in some of their patients, as well. I and others in the field have noticed that there is one neurological test in particular that many adults whose blood mercury level is higher than 20 mcg/l have difficulty performing. This is patterned sequential movements such as pat-a-cake, even though they knew how to do it. This resolves after blood mercury is reduced to less than 5 mcg/l.

When having any symptoms that are persistent or bothersome, patients need to be in the hands of a good internal medicine or family practitioner (primary care physician) who will investigate all causes, as mercury is a diagnosis of exclusion. Over the last eight years, I have diagnosed many other conditions in people who thought mercury was causing their problem. In some of these cases, whether mercury contributed was a moot point, as the mercury side effects can mostly be resolved by stopping consumption, while a cancer or other serious condition will not be cured just because you stopped consuming mercury. Sometimes patients can have symptoms of mercury side effects *and* a serious condition. As I mentioned earlier, the point at which lesser symptoms will lead to permanent damage is unknown at this time. For healthy living, I encourage all my patients to eat a balanced diet that includes fruits, vegetables, nuts and seeds, and healthy omega-3 choices and avoid processed foods with artificial ingredients. I also suggest pleasant exercise and medications only when indicated. For those at risk, I monitor the methylmercury intake through dietary recall and blood or hair analysis. Stress reduction and adequate sleep are emphasized, as well.

One of the biggest dilemmas in the realm of health effects of fish contaminants is the possible tradeoff between the contribution of methylmercury to increased risk of heart problems compared to the benefits of omega-3 fatty acids. The best review of the literature on evidence of this health threat so far comes from an ongoing study of Finnish men. Researchers showed that men with mercury levels in their hair of 2.03 mcg/g and greater (equivalent to about 8 mcg/l in whole blood) had an increased risk of heart disease, heart attack, and risk of death by about 1.6 times compared to those with hair mercury levels of less than 2.03 mcg/g. Those with the lowest mercury levels and with an elevated level of the good omega-3 fats in their blood had the least risk of heart disease.[10]

When I began looking at the cardiac studies and methylmercury human epidemiologic studies, I was especially curious about the cardiovascular disease risk of people in the Faroes and Seychelles. The Seychelles diet contained fish with mercury at a level that gave them the distinction of being one of the most methylmercury-exposed populations in the world. Cardiovascular disease was the number one killer in the Seychelles and accounted for 41 percent of all mortality. Of course, there could be a number of reasons for that, as there were multiple risk factors for heart disease, such as obesity, hypertension, diabetes, and smoking, evident in the population. I have not seen any published reports on methylmercury and heart disease in the Seychelles, however.[11] It is interesting to note that the Faroese also have considerable heart disease risk, but their morbidity and mortality have declined in the last eight years—as have their mercury levels. In 2001, the risk of death from cardiovascular disease among the Faroese was 40 percent. In the United States, heart disease accounted for 29 percent of all deaths. A high heart disease rate in populations that consume a lot of fish and methylmercury does not lend support to the notion that the benefits of omega-3 fatty acids outweigh the risk of methylmercury.[12]

The American Heart Association currently recommends that the average person eat a variety of preferably oily fish at least twice a week, as well as oils and other foods rich in alpha linolenic acid, such as flaxseed, canola, and soybean oils, and walnuts. For those with documented coronary heart disease, an intake of 1,000 mg per day of omega-3 fatty acids, eicosapentaenoic acid and docosahexaenoic acid (EPA/DHA), either as fatty fish or as supplements, is recommended as of this writing. According to the mercury and omega charts provided by the AHA and the Environmental Protection Agency, however, it would take twelve ounces of light tuna or four ounces of white tuna to give an individual 1,000 mg of EPA/DHA. The mercury content, though, would then be higher than 30 mcg/day, which in turn could raise the risk of heart disease. A person who consumed 2 to 3 ounces of wild salmon or sardines instead could get the omega-3 fatty acids with about ten times less methylmercury. Two ounces per day of herring or wild salmon would not be expected to raise a person's blood mercury over 5 mcg/l.[13]

Other non-fish sources of omega-3 fatty acids are some types of pigs, flax-fed chickens and their eggs, milk with an omega-3 supplement additive, and grass-fed beef. My undergraduate alma mater of California State University at Chico recently tested the fat content of beef fed with grain only, a grain and grass combination, and grass only. The grass-only diet significantly lowered the saturated fatty acid and raised the omega-3 fatty acid content in the meat by 40 percent. Competition in sources of supply will be a healthy addition to the omega-3 discussion.[14]

For those who prefer supplements for omega-3s, the supplement industry has made efforts to distill out the contaminants and purify the EPA/DHA product. Your supplement label should state that it has been tested for the content of contaminants and EPA/DHA. Omega-3 fatty acids in supplement form with concomitant use of aspirin (antiplatelet drugs) or coumadin or heparin (anticoagulant drugs) is currently not known. Since these combinations can potentially increase bleeding in the body, I recommend that you check with your doctor before you begin or stop your supplements.[15]

Variety is the key. I cannot stress this enough. No one should be consuming either salmon or tuna every day, so mix it up. Rotate your poisons. Eat your fruits and vegetables. Beyond that general advice, your consumption patterns, the type of fish caught or purchased, and circumstances such as your reproductive status and concurrent health should all be taken into consideration. The more fish one consumes, the lower in contaminants one would want it to be. Those who desire to consume fish every day need to be particularly diligent in educating themselves on mercury levels and other contaminants in different kinds of fish in their area. Even as recently as November 2006, I had a physician in his sixties consult me about his own blood mercury level of 25 mcg/l who knew nothing about any advisory from EPA, FDA, AHA, NAS, ATSDR, or a host of other acronymic agencies. He was suffering from fatigue, memory loss, tremor, and generalized ill feeling that had been waxing and waning for months. He had increased his canned tuna consumption to lose weight. Since the discovery that his problem could be related to his intake of methylmercury, he became diligent at keeping his mercury blood levels less than 5 mcg/l. At his one-year followup, he was doing well.

Should you want to estimate your likely methylmercury intake, here is some information that might be helpful. In calculating your own exposure to methylmercury using the FDA tables on the Web, it is important to know that the ranges of mercury level in the fish are not true ranges. It was recently disclosed by the FDA that each test they conducted was actually on a blended mixture of twelve different fish. The average, therefore, is an average of averages, and the highest number given in the range is lower than if individual fish were tested each time. Some nongovernment groups have been assisting the public in these calculations. Web sites such as http://gotmercury.org provide useful tools for those who want to continue to enjoy fish and maintain their mercury level at less than 5 mcg/l. Hopefully, more information on PCB levels will also become readily available.

To make sense of the FDA lists of fish with their mercury levels when you go to a grocery store or restaurant, there are several cautions needed. Restaurants will sometimes substitute one fish for another, and there is no regulation against it. This substitution is usually based on taste and availability and without consideration of the amount of mercury or PCBs in the substitution. Be sure you do not confuse the size of the portion with the size of the fish. The steak fish, such as tuna, halibut, and swordfish, are only a small piece of a large fish. Consider also that the common names of fish can change depending on the region where they are sold.

In choosing fish, as mentioned before, it is the large predatory fish such as swordfish, shark, king mackerel, tilefish, large tuna, sailfish, sea bass, grouper, pike, and large halibut that are usually longer lived, more predacious, and contain more mercury. They can also sometimes accumulate PCBs. Essentially, the smaller fatty fish, such as sardines, small mackerel, herring, anchovies, and salmon, are higher in omega-3 fatty acids but can be higher in PCBs and other contaminants, as well. These contaminants are contained more in the skin and fat; therefore, letting the juices flow out when you cook them and not eating the skin or fat can reduce your exposure. Methylmercury, on the other hand, is mostly in the muscle tissue, and no cooking methods have been shown to cook it out of the fish.[16] For noncommercial game fish, you need to consult your state Department of Fish and Game or the Web to check for the latest testing and advisories in the water body you are going to fish. The best way to assess your exposure is by assessing your dose. There is no way to tell just how much mercury you really have in your system, especially since some organs such as kidney, liver, brain, muscle, gastrointestinal tract, and heart tissue can have varying concentrations within the same body. Testing the mercury level in your hair will let you know your average excretion in the hair over a month's time of consumption, however. Hair grows about one centimeter per month on average, and mercury is strongly bound in hair. It cannot be washed out. You can check the mercury level at various lengths of your hair; hair will record the levels over time like rings on a tree. (How and whether permanents, straighteners, or dyes affect the hair mercury levels is currently not clearly known.) A blood level will give you a "spot check" and reflects both recent diet and accumulation.

~•~

The "nuanced" and "targeted" approach of the FDA's mercury warning system has left many consumers at risk for the contaminants of fish such as mercury and PCBs. The agency's 1 mcg/g methylmercury-in-fish action level is not adequate and not enforced, and it was derived using data that was flawed as well as misrepresented, as we've seen.

The EPA went beyond the action level in fish and identified a tolerable blood limit for mercury in humans and determined a dose that corresponds to that limit. The FDA, unfortunately, has still not fully embraced the EPA's human limit for mercury. Whether this human limit is protective for adults and the most sensitive individuals for long-term exposure will continue to be debated, considering the cardiac literature, but adoption of that standard by the FDA would be a move in the right direction.

The government agencies could do much to involve practicing clinicians in the mercury debate and in discussions over other potentially harmful chemicals to bridge the gap between public health policy and the individual patient. Physicians routinely discuss behavior and risk with individuals. My patients come to my office with their computers in hand. They have access to information just as we do. We as physicians and health care associates need to be there to let the public know how to navigate the information highway and analyze the data so that they can make informed decisions about their health. But there is something wrong with the system when a serious problem with a food item is evident enough that it gains warnings from the FDA, yet physicians across the nation, from the private doctor's office to the American Medical Association, typically do not know much if anything about it.

Confusion over the health effects of mercury is but one example of what happens when money, power, politics, and health collide over a pollutant. Because physicians were unaware of mercury's relatively low-dose health effects and how to recognize and address them, no case reports from physicians were being filed with the FDA. In turn, the FDA did not see the need to warn physicians and the public and concluded that there was no one in the United States eating enough fish to cause adverse effects from mercury. Our government agencies are inundated with not only the monitoring of food, drugs, and the environment, but also with pressure from industry, special interest groups, and nongovernment organizations, all with a stake in the final ruling. For the medical establishment to play an effective role in these decisions that ultimately affect our patients' health, environmental medicine and nutrition need to become part of a medical school education. The health care team needs to be involved in understanding environmental issues, learning how those issues may affect the health of patients, and bringing the importance of environmental factors to wider attention when we see their significance at the front lines.

People in medicine have an important role to play, but to cope with the range of issues surrounding pollutants such as mercury, it takes public awareness and concern, reform of the regulatory process, scientific investigation free of outside influence, and willingness of industry to take some action for the common good. None of us can possibly know everything. But there's much we can discover from mercury's history and effects on its victims, and from listening to each other.

Notes

Chapter 1. The Discovery

1. Wyngaarden 1992.
2. Mahaffey 1997.

Chapter 2. Finding My Way

1. Knobeloch 1995.
2. This is if the albacore had an average mercury level of 0.36 mcg/g. This is because the 60-kg person is allowed up to 42 mcg/week, and 114 g of albacore that is 0.36 mcg/g would be about 41.4 mcg of mercury. I also realized that there was no uniform or user-friendly standard of laboratory reporting for mercury. Some labs used parts per million (ppm) for mcg/g and parts per billion (ppb) for mcg/l. When the same lab reported in mcg/l one day and mcg/deciliter (dl) another, this especially became confusing and led to physician and patient errors in interpretation of the results. I urged the media to use mcg/l and mcg/g as the units of measure, so that everyone could understand, compare, and interpret the results. What is a "part," anyway? I do not know how to do math on a part. Using parts as a measure seemed like going back to tinctures and grains for medications.
3. U.S. Food and Drug Administration 1995.

Chapter 3. The Media Meets the Victims

1. Pam Moore, interview for KRON *Channel 4 News*, San Francisco, August 2, 2000; story aired August 3, 2000.
2. Patricia Steele, personal communication by phone, 2000.

Chapter 4. Spreading the News

1. J. M. Hightower to Senator Dianne Feinstein, August 17, 2000.
2. D. Feinstein to Ms. Diane E. Thompson, September 27, 2000, www.cfsan.fda.gov/~acrobat/hgcong73.pdf.
3. M. Plaisier to the Honorable Dianne Feinstein, undated, received December 21, 2000, www.cfsan.fda.gov/~acrobat/hgcong74.pdf.
4. Myers 1995, main neurodevelopmental study; Marsh 1995, Seychelles Study; Grandjean 1998.

5. National Academy of Sciences 2000.

6. Mahaffey 1997.

7. "The Fish Risk," *20/20*, January 12, 2001.

8. Public Health Service 1993. Highlights of the report.

9. Ibid.

10. Nightingale 1991; American Dental Association 1991; Truono 1991; Mezei 1990.

11. Public Health Service 1993.

Chapter 5. A Spoonful of Mercury

1. "The Story of the Laws behind the Labels: Part I, 1906 Food and Drugs Act" 1981.

2. "The Story of the Laws behind the Labels: Part II, 1938—The Federal Food, Drug, and Cosmetic Act" 1981.

3. "The Story of the Laws behind the Labels: Part III, 1962 Drug Amendments" 1981.

4. Goldwater 1972; D'Itri 1977.

5. Goldwater 1972, p. 25.

6. Rhead 1895; Sexton 1899.

7. Goldwater 1972; D'Itri 1977.

8. Grun 1982; Hirschhorn 2001; Corish 1927.

9. Clendening 1942.

10. Goldwater 1972.

11. Ibid.

12. Transactions of the American Medical Association 1864; Brieger 1967; Flannery 2004.

13. American Medical Association 1864, p. 31.

14. American Medical Association 1864, pp. 32–33

15. Brieger 1967; Flannery 2004.

16. Hirschhorn 2001; Flannery 2004.

17. Vogl 1950.

18. DeGraff 1942, pp. 998–1001; Barker 1942; Brown 1942; DeGraff 1942, pp. 1006–1011. All of these are from *JAMA*, 119(13). Also see Greiner 1953.

19. World Health Organization 1972.

20. DeGraff 1942 and DeGraff 1942; American Pharmaceutical Association 1950; Howard 1952.

21. De Forest 1944; De Forest 1949; Stanford University School of Medicine 1959.

22. American Pharmaceutical Association 1950; Howard 1952; Brewer 1939; Morton 1948.

23. O'Carroll 1995; Dinehart 1988.

24. U.S. Food and Drug Administration, Department of Health and Human Services, April 22, 1998; December 14, 1998; Howard 1952; American Pharmaceutical Association 1950; Brewer 1939.

25. Hyson 2006, p. 216.

26. Spaeth 2002; Dye 2005; Hyson 2006.

27. Hyson 2006, p. 217.

28. Hyson 2006, p. 219

29. Ibid.

30. Ibid., p. 225.

31. Valentine-Thon 2003; Stejskal 1999; Stejskal 1999.

32. U.S. Patent and Trademark Office 1928.

33. Powell 1931; Jamieson 1931; Powell 1932; Powell 1938.

34. Rosenstein 1935; Morton 1948; Falk 1936; Mortensen 1954; Haggerty 1960.

35. Pichichero 2002, p. 1741.

36. University of Rochester Medical Center 2007; Pichichero 2000; Pichichero 2005.

37. Pichichero 2008, p. e214

38. Geier 2003; Geier 2003; Geier 2006.

39. U.S. Food and Drug Administration letter to vaccine manufacturers 1999.

40. Bassler 1935; LeBlanc 1936.

41. Newschaffer 2007.

42. Guy 1923; Puckner 1932; Rajakumar 2003; Murphy 2001.

Chapter 6. Making Money with a Menace

1. Ramazzini 1713.

2. O'Carroll 1995; Neal 1937; Neal 1941. The latter reports were obtained from the Environmental Protection Agency and detail the hatter investigation by the Public Health Department.

3. Committee Minutes, Hat Makers and Hat Finishers Locals no. 10 and 11, May 5, 1951.

4. Varekamp 2003.

5. Goldwater 1972.

6. Christopher Columbus letter to the king and queen of Spain 1490s; Marcus 1938.

7. Smith 1995. The Emanuel Point Ship, wrecked off the Florida Coast, contained some flasks of quicksilver.

8. Goldwater 1972.

9. Stern 1982.

10. Davies 1996; Goldwater 1972.

11. Personal communication with Tracy Bowden, treasure diver, 2004.

12. Stevenson 2002.

13. Tracy Bowden, personal communication, 2004. Bowden has the salvage rights to these ships. He can be seen in a 1972 *National Geographic* pouring quicksilver in a pan while under water. When I first called him, he immediately asked if I were "leadin' some sort of movement." He subsequently was a delight in speaking of the old shipwrecks of the sea.

14. Of her 650 passengers, 550 managed to reach shore, but one lifeboat with 240 passengers drifted for days until reaching Cap Hatien 240 miles away. Starving and exhausted, many died shortly thereafter.

15. Putman 1972; personal communication with Roy Roush, PhD, professor and treasure diver, 2004. It was noted that emblems from the Knights of Santiago were found in the wreckage. Further reading about this order can be found in Sainty, *The Spanish Military Orders* (2004) and *The Military Order of Santiago* (2004).

16. Some treasure divers have speculated that much of the four hundred tons spilled in the Dominican Republic appears to be there still under the shallow sand. They said it would take a meeting of the nations to clean it up.

17. Bedoya 2001; Grandjean 1999; Ortiz-Roque 2004; Olivero 2002; Adams 2004.

18. Mahaffey 1997.

19. U.S. Environmental Protection Agency 2003. Page 70920 contains the "enigma" statement made by the EPA; American Medical Association 2006.

20. Smith 1975; D'Itri 1977. Much of the information comes from these two books. The Smiths and the D'Itris were very diligent in following the mercury issues of Canada, United States, and Japan in the 1970s.

21. Ibid. The famous cat #400 experiment is best described in the Smith book. Excerpts from Dr. Hosokawa's testimony are printed on p. 122. Eugene describes his beating as the Goi incident (pp. 94–95).

22. Ibid.

23. T. Tsuda, personal correspondence, 2007; Tsuda 2006. Dr. Tsuda has a page on Aileen Smith's Web site, http://aileenarchive.or.jp/minamata_en/testimonials/index.html. Also see Futatsuka 2005.

24. Aileen Smith, personal communication, November 2007.

25. Smith 1975; D'Itri 1977; Harada 1978; Igata 1993; Harada 1995; Fukuda 1999; Ekino 2007.

26. Associated Press 2004.

27. *Japan Times* 2004.

28. Associated Press 2004.

29. Mahaffey 1997; U.S. Environmental Protection Agency 2008.

30. Scorecard 2008

31. Riley 2001; Prasad 2004.

Chapter 7. The Summit

1. Hightower 2001.
2. Mahaffey 1997.
3. Hightower and Moore April 2003. Hair levels of mercury among the seven tested in this way ranged from 1.55 to 14.81 mcg/g.
4. Ibid.

Chapter 8. Feeling the Heat in Mercury Politics

1. Mahaffey 1997.
2. U.S. Court of Appeals 2008; U.S. Food and Drug Administration 2001.
3. U.S. Food and Drug Administration 1995.
4. Hightower to Senator Dianne Feinstein, November 20, 2002.
5. Salonen 1995; Rissanen 2000; Guallar 2002.
6. Hightower and Mates 2003, Resolution 112-03.
7. California Department of Justice 2003.
8. CMA 2003.
9. Davidson 2003.
10. Rickey 1998.
11. American Medical Association 2004.
12. JIFSAN 1998–1999.
13. Myers 2003; Clarkson 2003; Myers 1997.
14. These were statements that Lyketsos and Myers allegedly sent to the *Lancet*. They were forwarded to me by Linda Greer and Jennifer Sass.
15. The first paper was entitled "Verification of Techniques for Assessing the Effects of Methylmercury and Other Neurotoxicants on Neurodevelopment in Children." The second was entitled "Prenatal Methylmercury Exposure from Ocean Fish Consumption in the Seychelles Child Development Study."
16. Crump 2000.
17. Davidson 2003; Clarkson 2003; Myers 2003.
18. Fialka 2003.

Chapter 9. The Canadian Mercury Scare

1. D'Itri 1977; Personal communication by phone with F. D'Itri 2003, 2006; Smith 1975.
2. D'Itri 1977.
3. D'Itri 1977; CBC November 6, 1974.
4. Ibid.
5. Ibid.
6. D'Itri 1977; CBC November 6, 1974; November 7, 1974.

7. D'Itri 1977; CBC November 6, 1974; Ontario Department of Health 1972.

8. D'Itri 1977.

9. The Marion Lamm Collection at Harvard's Environmental Science and Public Policy archive is the largest collection of documents relating to the Canadian mercury problem from 1969 through the 1980s.

10. Ontario Department of Health 1972.

11. Ontario Legislature 1974.

12. International Joint Commission 2007.

13. Mackenzie 2005; Environment Canada 2007.   .

14. D'Itri 1977; CBC November 6, 1974; November 7, 1974.

15. Ibid.

16. D'Itri 1977; CBC November 1, 1970; November 7, 1974; August 20, 1975; September 23, 1975; January 14, 1976; March 15, 1983.

17. Takeuchi 1977.

18. Smith 1975; D'Itri 1977.

19. Clarkson and Shapiro 1971; Clarkson and Small 1971; CBC September 23, 1975.

20. Ibid.

21. Smith 1975; D'Itri 1977.

22. CBC September 23, 1975.

23. Harada 1976; D'Itri 1977; CBC September 23, 1975.

24. CBC August 20, 1975.

25. Smith 1975; D'Itri 1977; CBC August 20, 1975; September 29, 1975.

26. CBC November 7, 1974.

27. Ibid.

28. Ibid.

29. Ibid.

30. CBC November 7, 1974; September 29, 1975.

31. CBC September 29, 1975.

32. Clarkson and Shapiro 1971; Clarkson and Small 1971, 1976. Clarkson worked on his Dow resin and reported his findings as late as 1981. He had also developed the most accurate mercury testing procedure and machine at the time.

33. Wheatley 1979.

34. Ibid

35. D'Itri 1977.

36. Ibid.

37. Ibid.

38. Ibid. Fishmeal, often used for animal chow, was also of concern, as mercury was discovered to concentrate in the course of processing fishmeal more

than five times higher than in fresh fish. For example, the mercury content of carp—0.58 mcg/g fresh—concentrated to 3.12 mcg/g in fishmeal.

39. D'Itri 1977, p. 59
40. D'Itri 1977.
41. Harada 2005.
42. World Health Organization 1990.
43. CBC November 25, 1985; Hechtman 2003; Mackenzie 2005.
44. CBC November 7, 1974.
45. Creber 2003; Schabath 2002.

Chapter 10. Dr. Sa'adoun al-Tikriti

1. Kunin 1989.
2. U.S. Food and Drug Administration July 2003.
3. Smith 1975; D'Itri 1977.
4. U.S. Environmental Protection Agency 1999.
5. Smith 1975; D'Itri 1977; Mahaffey 1997.
6. Bakir 1973.
7. Thamery, personal communication in San Francisco, 2004.
8. Tikriti, personal communication by phone, 2004.

Chapter 11. Fishy Loaves

1. World Health Organization 2000, 2004.
2. D'Itri 1977, pp. 31, 37, 45.
3. Bakir 1973.
4. This WHO report was later mentioned in the book in a court trial and has been mentioned in other WHO reports. To date, I have been unable to obtain a copy of it.
5. D'Itri 1977, p. 37; D'Itri F., personal communication by phone 2003; 2006.
6. Hughes 1973. Hughes 1973. Both the *London Sunday Times* and *Reader's Digest* are variations of his report.
7. Amin-Zaki 1986.
8. Hughes 1973. *London Sunday Times.*
9. Cargill 2004; Cargill Switzerland 2004; Sutton 1997. By 1997, Cargill was one of the largest salt production and marketing companies in the world.
10. Cargill 2004; Cargill Switzerland 2004.
11. Hughes 1973 and 1973; Damluji 1962; Al-Kassab 1962; Haq 1963; Dahan 1964.
12. Bakir 1973. See pp. 231 and 236.
13. Tikriti, personal communication, 2004.
14. Futatsuka 2005; Ekino 2007.

15. Giles 2003.

16. Damluji and Tikriti 1972.

17. Hughes 1973. *London Sunday Times*; Bakir 1973.

18. Bakir 1973; D'Itri 1977; Giles 2003.

19. Clarkson and Shapiro 1971, Clarkson and Smith 1971, Clarkson 1973, 1981; D'Itri 1977.

20. Clarkson and Shapiro 1971. The first lecture I could find by Clarkson on his Dow resin was "The Absorption of Mercury from Food: Its Significance and New Methods of Removing Mercury from the Body," delivered in February 1971 at a Royal Society of Canada symposium.

21. Al Kassab 1962, p. 118.

22. Miller 1990; Karsh 1991; Aburish 2000; Coughlin 2002; Munthe 2002. I used multiple history texts to gather information on Saddam and the history of Iraq.

23. Aburish 2000, p. 61.

24. Coughlin 2002, p. 43

25. Graham 2003.

26. Coughlin 2002.

27. Aburish 2000, p. 80.

28. Coughlin 2002. According to Coughlin, just before the takeover of the country, Saddam decreed that "Those deemed enemies of the party were to be killed. Unfriendly factions intimidated." He was known to "love to hurt." In January 5, 1969, seventeen "spies" went on trial; fourteen were hung, eleven of them Jewish. Bakr's and Saddam's series of "purges [were] designed to eliminate opposition to the government."

29. Miller 1990; Karsh 1991; Aburish 2000; Coughlin 2002; Munthe 2002.

30. Bakir 1973.

31. Bakir 1976.

32. Amin-Zaki 1986; also personal communications with Dr. Thamery and Dr. Tikriti. Dr. Damluji, of the University of Baghdad, who wrote papers about the 1960 poisoning well into 1964, together with his wife, Laman Amin-Zaki, investigated the 1971–1972 poisonings, and indicated that there were no reports of mercury seed grain poisonings in Iraq between 1960 and 1971.

33. Bakir 1973, p. 232.

34. Hughes 1973 and 1973.

35. Ibid.

36. Ibid.

37. Hughes 1973. *London Sunday Times*, p. 17

38. Hughes 1973 and 1973; D'Itri 1977.

39. Hughes 1973. *London Sunday Times*, p. 19.

40. Clarkson 1981.

41. Hughes 1973 and 1973; D'Itri 1977.

42. Hughes 1973 and 1973; Bakir 1973.

43, Hughes 1973. *London Sunday Times*, p. 19.

44. "Mercury in the Environment" 1972.

45. Miller 1990; Karsh 1991; Aburish 2000; Coughlin 2002; Munthe 2002.

46. Ibid.

47. Karsh 1991, pp. 72–73

48. *World Culture Encyclopedia* 2007.

49. Coughlin 2002.

50. Ibid. All four chemicals were precursors to nerve gas agents. Pfaudler representatives did not give in to this full-scale plant, but they provided specifics that would enable Iraq to build its own plant.

Chapter 12. Fishing with the FDA for Evidence in Iraq

1. *British Medical Journal* 1972; Damluji 1972.

2. Bakir 1973; Amin-Zaki 1974, p. 590.3. Amin-Zaki 1978.

4. Grandjean, personal communication by e-mail, October 2004.

5. *United States of America vs. Anderson Seafoods, Inc.*, judge's opinion, 1978; *United States of America vs. Anderson Seafoods, Inc.*, trial, August 16–18, 1977.

6. Ibid.

7. Ibid.

8. The FDA, industry, and WHO considered the average weight of an individual to be about 60 kilograms, or 132 pounds. If a person of average weight consumed 30 mcg of mercury per day, he or she would have a blood level of about 22.5 mcg/l. At a dose of 300 mcg/day, a person's blood would be about 225 mcg/l.

9. Albacore tuna has been measured to be on average 0.3–0.5 mcg/g, depending on the study.

10. *United States of America vs. Anderson Seafoods, Inc.*, August 16, 1977.

Chapter 13. Fishing with the Industry for Evidence in Iraq

1. *United States of America vs. Anderson Seafoods, Inc.*, 1978.

2. It was unclear from his testimony how much methylmercury was consumed by the rats that were fed swordfish.

3. *United States of America vs. Anderson Seafoods, Inc.*, August 17 transcript, p. 599. Blumberg showed Friedman a report by the Rochester researchers, who included David Marsh and Thomas Clarkson, that stated

the dose-response data from Iraq to determine the critical level of methyl-mercury toxicity for humans have been inadequate.

4. *United States of America vs. Anderson Seafoods, Inc.* August 17, p. 606

5. Ibid., pp. 610, 624.

6. Ibid, p. 615.

7. Ibid., pp. 667, 691, 692, 698.

8. Ibid., pp. 713, 715.

9. Ibid., p. 723.

10. Ibid., pp. 726, 744, 745.

11. Bakir 1973, p. 240. Tikriti, personal communication 2004.

12. *United States of America Vs Anderson Seafoods, Inc.* August 17 transcript. Industry lawyer Robert Lasky quickly allowed Crispin-Smith to reinforce his Iraqi data calculations by asking about studies in Samoa and Peru. Crispin-Smith claimed "that there was no evidence in these populations that any signs or symptoms that could be attributed to ingestion of methylmercury in fish could be found"; p. 722.

13. Ibid., p. 749; this was using a safety factor of 5 (120 mcg/day). His conclusions were similar to Friedman's, except that instead of a no-observable-effect level, Crispin-Smith compromised and used the minimal-clinical-effect level.

14. Ibid., pp. 756–761.

15. Ibid., p. 768.

16. Ibid., pp. 777–784, 794–811.

17. Ibid.

18. Ibid., pp. 817–81

19. Ibid. Dr. Margolin's testimony is on pp. 866–911.

20. Ibid., p. 926

21. Ibid. Dr. Marsh's testimony is on pp. 911–939. "Minimal effects" quote on pp. 923–24.

22. Ibid., p. 930.

23. The original trial date was set for July 18, 1977. Clarkson could not be there due to another commitment, so it was decided that a deposition would take place in June. Clarkson then stated that he was able to reschedule his July engagement to September; therefore, he would be at the trial. The trial got moved to August 15–18, 1977, and Clarkson again said he could not be there because of a prior commitment. The judge then said that the testimony of Dr. Clarkson in the court could take place on September 21 and ordered it to be done then. Unfortunately, this was when Clarkson had rescheduled his previous engagement in order to attend the July trial date. At that point, the FDA had three choices: Force Clarkson to alter his plans for a third time by

subpoenaing him to court, dispense with his testimony entirely, or take his deposition after the trial.

24. Ibid. Motion to prohibit filing of Dr. Clarkson's deposition unless filed under seal; memorandum in support of motion to prohibit filing of deposition; government's memorandum in reply; government's memorandum in support of opposition to require sealing of deposition; Anderson Seafoods memorandum in opposition to government's motion for leave; government's motion in opposition to require sealing the deposition of Dr. Clarkson; judge's ruling on the sealing of the deposition.

25. Ibid., the deposition of Thomas Clarkson, September 17, 1977.

26. Bakir 1973, p. 237

27. Ibid., *United States of America vs. Anderson Seafoods, Inc.* August 18 transcript, pp. 861–62. Her name was spelled Bettye Russow in the published scientific paper that presented her case. The D'Itris' book provided the proper spelling.

28. Korns 1972; D'Itri 1977, pp. 64–65. The D'Itris stated in their book that she was on a Weight Watchers program.

29. *United States of America vs. Anderson Seafoods, Inc.* The Deposition of Thomas Clarkson, September 17, 1977, p. 100

30. Ibid., p. 97

31. Marsh 1980.

32. Bakir 1980.

33. Marsh 1987.

34. Giles 2003.

35. Watson 2002; Giles 2003; Stone 2003; Curtis 2003.

Chapter 14. From American Samoa to Peru

1. Turner 1974, 1980; Marsh 1974; Marsh 1995, Fetal methylmercury study in a Peruvian fish-eating population; Myers 2000.

2. *United States of America vs. Anderson Seafoods, Inc.*, August 18 transcript, p. 930.

3. Marsh 1974. Grants came from the Tuna Research Foundation as well as the National Science Foundation, the National Institute of Arthritis, Metabolism and Digestive Diseases, the National Institute of General Medical Sciences, the National Institute of Neurological Disorders and Stroke.

4. Darden 1951.

5. Purcell International 2008; Faleomavaega May 2003; Chicken of the Sea 2008.

6. Marsh 1974; Hightower and Moore 2003.

7. Faleomavaega May 2003.

8. Gillet 2004; Australian Government 2004; U.S. Department of Labor 2005; U.S. Department of State 2004, Samoa; Faleomavaega May 2003; June 16, 2003; June 19, 2003.

9. Ibid.

10. Putman 1972.

11. IDDRA 2004.

12. NOAA Fisheries 2004.

13. Turner 1974, 1980.

14. Turner 1974, 1980; Marsh 1995, Fetal methylmercury study in a Peruvian fish-eating population.

15. Turner 1974, 1980. The twelve signs listed as methylmercury-related were diminished ankle reflexes, mental retardation, eczema, impaired peripheral touch, reduced ankle vibration sense, impaired hearing, ataxic gait, dementia, ataxia of limbs, impaired perioral sensation, visual field constriction, and dysarthria. The fourteen symptoms were distal limb paresthesia, impaired vision, impaired hearing, headache, perioral paresthesia, tremor, poor memory, mental retardation, anorexia and weight loss, epilepsy, impaired peripheral vision, ataxia of gait, ataxia of limbs, and slurred speech.

16. Marsh 1995, Fetal methylmercury study in a Peruvian fish-eating population; they studied 131 mother-infant pairs in Mancora, where they found peak maternal hair methylmercury concentrations during pregnancy from 1.2 mcg/g to 30 mcg/g with a mean of 8.34 mcg/g (30 mcg/g of hair would be approximately 120 mcg/l blood). The survey began at a fishing port, where they took hair samples of pregnant women, many of whom were fishermen's wives. Other areas were surveyed, as well.

17. Lewis 1997.

18. Appenzeller 2002; U.S. Sentencing Commission 1995.

19. The total mercury level is the level of all the mercury compounds, such as elemental mercury and methylmercury, combined. The machine used to quantitate the total mercury level heats the specimen to extremely high temperatures, so that all the carbon atoms are removed. The remaining mercury is what is quantitated.

20. Turner 1980.

Chapter 15. The Political Realm of Seychelles versus Faroes

1. Children's Health and the Environment in the Faroes 2004; Fishinfo 2006; *Marine Fisheries Review* 1989; U.S. Department of State, Denmark 2004; Hites 2004.

2. Grandjean 1994, 1998; Debes 2006; Sørensen 1999; Murata 2004. The tests included the Neurobehavioral Evaluation System finger-tapping test,

hand-eye coordination test, and continuous performance test (a test for attention span); the Weschler Intelligence Scale for Children–Revised digit spans, similarities, and block design tests; the Bender Visual Motor Gestalt Test; California Verbal Learning Test; and the Boston Naming Test.

3. Grandjean 1994, 1998; Debes 2006; Sørensen 1999; Murata 2004.

4. Ibid.

5. Mahaffey 2005.

6. Sørensen 1999; Murata 2004.

7. Budtz-Jørgensen 2007.

8. Matthews 1983; Poulter 2007.

9. Myers 1995, "Pilot Neurodevelopmental Study"; Marsh 1995, "The Seychelles Study."

10. Davidson 2000. The tests given were the Wechsler Intelligence Test for Children–III, the California Verbal Learning Test, the Boston Naming Test, the Beery-Buktenica Developmental Test of Visual-Motor Integration, the Wide Range Assessment of Memory and Learning, the Grooved Pegboard Dexterity Test, the Trail Making Test (of speed of visual search), and the finger-tapping test. Only the grooved pegboard showed a decrease in performance with increased cord blood levels.

11. Myers 1995, "Main Neurodevelopmental Study"; Marsh 1995, "The Seychelles Study." The tests given to the infants were the Denver Developmental Screening Test–Revised, a basic neurological exam; Fagan's test of visual recognition memory (Infatest); the Bayley Scales of Infant Development (tests psychomotor and mental development), and the McCarthy Scales of Children's Abilities (tests cognitive function). From the graph given in the report, all mothers were under 30 mcg/g, and less than 3 percent were in the 20–25 mcg/g range—about 34 percent were greater than 10 mcg/g.

12. Myers 2003, *Lancet*.

13. Crump 2000.

14. Myers 1995, "Main Neurodevelopmental Study."

15. Ibid.

16. Ibid.

17. Shamlaye 1995.

18. U.S. Department of State 2004, "Background Note: Seychelles."

19. International Trade Centre 1999; UK Trade and Investment 2004.

20. International Trade Centre 1999.

21. Ibid.

22. Gillett 2004.

23. Clarkson 2000; Archer 2001.

24. Wijngaarden 2006.

25. Personal communication with Grandjean, May 2007.

26. Wijngaarden 2006.

Chapter 16. The Mercury Study Report

1. U.S. Environmental Protection Agency, 2008, Clean Air Act 1986; U.S. Environmental Protection Agency, 2004, Clean Air Act Amendments of 1990.

2. Fitzgerald 1991.

3. Ibid.

4. Mahaffey 1997.

5. Egeland 1997.

6. Clarkson 1998.

7. Mahaffey 1997; National Academy of Sciences 2000; Mahaffey, personal communication by phone, 2001; U.S. Court of Appeals 2008.

8. Salonen 1995, 2000; Rissanen 2000; Guallar 2002; Virtanen 2005.

9. Burros 2001; American Heart Association 2002.

10. B. Clinton 2004; H. Clinton 2003; Hamilton 2003; Walker 1996.

11. B. Clinton 2004; H. Clinton 2003. It was Jim Blair who helped Hillary turn $1,000 into $100,000 in futures trading.

12. Walker 1996.

13. Tyson Foods, Inc. 2004; Egeland 1997.

14. Alaska Conservation Foundation 2000.

Chapter 17. Strategic Errors and Redundant Tactics

1. Canadian Press 1979; "Ohio Claims DOW, Wyandotte Knowingly Discharged Mercury" 1971; Crook 1971; Indian and Northern Affairs 2004.

2. *United States of America vs. Anderson Seafoods, Inc.* August 18. Marsh testimony, pp. 923–24.

3. Open Secrets 2004; Open Secrets 2005; Open Secrets 2005.

4. CDC 2001, 2004; National Center for Health Statistics 2005.

5. U.S. Environmental Protection Agency 2008, Clear Skies Act of 2003; U.S. Court of Appeals 2008.

6. CDC 2004.

7. Hightower 2006. We published our report in a peer-reviewed journal.

8. U.S. Tuna Foundation 2005; Pombo 2005.

9. Pombo 2005.

10. Pombo 2005; Keating 1997; Evers 2007.

11. Pombo 2005.

12. American Heart Association 2008. See the three Web sites that pertain to seafood endorsement programs, canned/pouch seafood, fresh seafood, and frozen seafood.

13. American Heart Association 2008, "Fish, Levels of Mercury and Omega-3 Fatty Acids."

14. Nesheim 2006.

15. Nesheim 2006.

16. Mozaffarian 2006.

17. Seppanen 2000; Mozaffarian 2006.

18. Nesheim 2006; Mozaffarian 2006.

19. U.S. Department of Agriculture, Food and Nutrition Service 2006.

20. Luke 2006.

21. U.S. Court of Appeals 2008.

Chapter 18. The Canning of Proposition 65 Mercury Warnings

1. *People of the State of California* 2006. Defendants proposed findings of fact and conclusions of law. Burney, 15 Tr:1790–1921. See especially pp. 1803, 1821, 1825, 1828, 1832

2. Ibid.

3. Ibid.

4. The canners declared that the State knew (1) that the tuna canners' compliance with Prop. 65 relied on averaging tuna consumption; (2) the average mercury concentrations in light and albacore tuna; (3) that canned tuna complied with the draft MADL (that relied on the Bornhausen rat study); and (4) the tuna canners' reasons for believing that methylmercury in tuna was naturally occurring.

5. Although I was invited and attended a meeting with the deputy AG, and did sign on to an amicus brief with the San Francisco Medical Society with others, I was never part of the actual trial. My "unordinary" people and I could therefore only sit and watch as the parade came through.

6. People of the State of California 2006. Findings of fact and conclusions of law re: preemption, MADL, and naturally occurring. April 17, 2006.

7. Ibid., pp. 6–9

8. Ibid.

9. Frustaci 1999; Guallar 2002; Rissanen 2000; Salonen 2000; Sørensen 1999; Virtanen 2005; Bagenstose 1999; Bernier 1995; Bigazzi 1994; Nielsen 2002; Silva 2004; Stejskal 1999, 1999; Via 2003; Choy 2002; Dickman 1998; Leung 2001; Sheiner 2003; Beuter 2004; Yokoo 2003; Fukuda 1999; Mergler 1998.

10. *People of the State of California* 2006. Findings of fact and conclusions of law re: preemption, MADL, and naturally occurring. April 17, 2006.

11. Ibid., p. 10.

12. *People of the State of California* 2006. Findings of fact and conclusions

of law re: preemption, MADL, and naturally occurring. April 17, 2006, p. 21; Bornhausen 1980.

13. Kraepiel 2003. Also, the final calculations by the industry experts were as follows: The FDA obtained an average methylmercury level for canned light tuna of 0.12 mcg/g and an average for canned albacore of 0.35 mcg/g. Dr. Murray derived a "weighted average" of methylmercury concentration for the combined canned light tuna and albacore of 0.239–0.257 mcg/g. For the finale, 0.239–0.257 mcg/g ×1 serving/60 days calculates out to be 0.26–0.28 mcg of mercury per day, and voila! The canned tuna are just below the MADL of the rat study of 0.3 mcg/d (NOEL of 300 mcg/d).

14. *People of the State of California* 2006. Findings of fact and conclusions of law re: preemption, MADL, and naturally occurring, pp. 58–69.

15. Ibid.

16. *People of the State of California* 2006. People's objections to court's proposed statement of decision.

17. *People of the State of California* 2006. People's objections to court's proposed statement of decision.

18. Personal communication with Philippe Grandjean by phone 2006. In 2007, Dr. Grandjean and his colleagues published a report that addressed the "confounders" such as PCBs in the mercury analysis data. The statistics showed that such confounders would cause the toxic effects of methylmercury to be underestimated—just the opposite of what the fishing industry had presented. See Budtz-Jørgensen 2007.

19. Ekstrom 2006; Mercury 2006.

20. Ibid.

Chapter 19. Diagnosis Mercury

1. Trasande 2005.

2. Smith 1975, pp. 7–8. Also, in an e-mail to me, Aileen Smith stated that Clarkson told them that they shouldn't bother going to Japan "because the incident was over." This was in the fall of 1970—Scientific Conference on Mercury at Rochester.

3. Smith, personal communication by email 2007.

4. Oken 2008.

5. Beuter 2004; Yokoo 2003; Fukuda 1999; Mergler 1998.

6. Sheiner 2003; Choy 2002; Leung 2001; Dickman 1998.

7. Silva 2004; Via 2003; Nielsen 2002; Stejskal 1999, 1999; Bagenstose 1999; Bernier 1995; Bigazzi 1994.

8. Fukuda 1999; Harada 1995, 2005.

9. Ibid.

10. Virtanen 2005; Sørensen 1999; Salonen 1995, 2000; Rissanen 2000; Guallar 2002; Frustaci 1999; Stern 2005.

11. Bovet 1997; Shamlaye 1995.

12. CDC 2008; Miljøministeriet 2003. AMAP Greenland and the Faroe Islands 1997–2001.

13. Kris-Etherton 2002; Mahaffey 2004; "Omega-3 Oil: Fish or Pills" 2003; Burger 2004, 2005, 2006; Storelli 2002; Morrissey 2004.

14. Daley 2005.

15. McClaskey 2007; Buckley 2004.

16. Hites 2004; Jacobs 2002; Mozaffarian 2006; Chicourel 2001; Morgan 1997; Ueno 2005.

Bibliography

Aburish, S. K. 2000. *Saddam Hussein: The Politics of Revenge*. London: Bloomsbury.

Adams, D. H. 2004. Total mercury levels in tunas from offshore waters of the Florida Atlantic Coast. *Marine Pollution Bulletin* 49(7–8): 659–63.

Agency for Toxic Substances and Disease Registry. 2001. Polychlorinated biphenyls. February. www.atsdr.cdc.gov/tfacts17.pdf.

Alaska Conservation Foundation. 2000. Toxic pollution in Alaska. *ACF Dispatch*. www.akcf.org. Summer.

Al-Kassab, S., and N. Saigh. 1962. Mercury and calcium excretion in chronic poisoning with organic mercury compounds. *J Fac Med Baghdad* 4(3): 118–23.

American Dental Association. 1991. American Dental Association statement on dental amalgam. *ASDC J Dent Child* 58(2): 88–89.

American Heart Association. 2002. The American Heart Association food certification program. www.starkist.com/nutrition/aha/aha.html.

———. 2008. The American Heart Association food certification program. Seafood: Canned/pouch seafood. www.checkmark.heart.org/AdCategory/SF/SF-CSF.

———. 2008. The American Heart Association food certification program. Seafood: Fresh seafood. www.checkmark.heart.org/AdCategory/SF/SF-ESF.

———. 2008. The American Heart Association food certification program. Seafood: Frozen seafood. www.checkmark.heart.org/AdCategory/SF/SF-OSF.

———. 2008. Fish, levels of mercury and omega-3 fatty acids. www.american heart.org/presenter.jhtml?identifier=3013797.

The American Medical Association. 1864. Comments on Surgeon General Circular #6. *Trans Am Med Assoc.* 14:29–33.

———. 2004. Report 13 of the Council on Scientific Affairs (A-04). Mercury and fish consumption: Medical and public health issues. Resolution 516 (A-03) (reference committee E). www.ama-assn.org/ama/pub/article/2036 -8669.html.

———. 2006. Report 1 of the Council on Science and Public Health (I-06). Mercury pollution. www.ama-assn.org/ama/pub/category/print/17010.html.

American Pharmaceutical Association. 1950. *The National Formulary*, 9th ed. Washington, DC: Author.

Amin-Zaki, L. 1986. A tale of two alkylmercury poisoning epidemics in Iraq. Report to the World Health Organization. This report was given to me by Dr. Philippe Grandjean of Harvard University in 2007.

Amin-Zaki, L., S. Elhassani, M. A. Majeed, T. W. Clarkson, R. A. Doherty, and M. Greenwood. 1974. Intra-uterine methylmercury poisoning in Iraq. *Pediatrics* 54(5): 587–95.

Amin-Zaki, L., M. A. Majeed, T. W. Clarkson, and M. R. Greenwood. 1978. Methylmercury poisoning in Iraqi children: Clinical observations over two years. *Brit Med J* 1: 613–16.

Appenzeller, O., P. K. Thomas, S. Posford, J. L. Gamboa, R. Caceda, and P. Milner. 2002. Acral paresthesias in the Andes and neurology at sea level. *Neurology* 59(10).

Archer, M. C., T. W. Clarkson, and J. J. Strain. 2001. Genetic aspects of nutrition and toxicology: Report of a workshop. *J Am College of Nutrition* 20(2): 119–28.

Associated Press (Kozo Mizoguchi). 2004. Japan's top court orders government to pay Minamata mercury poisoning victims 22 years after case filed. 15 October. http://staugustine.com/stories/101604/wor_2646156.shtml.

Australian Government, Department of Foreign Affairs and Trade. 2004. American Samoa Country Brief. September. www.dfat.gov.au/geo/american_samoa/american_samoa_brief.html.

Bagenstose, L. M., P. Salgame, and M. Monesteir. 1999. Murine mercury-induced autoimmunity: A model of chemically related autoimmunity in humans. *Immunologic Res* 20: 67–78.

Bakir, F., H. Al-Shahristani, N. Y. Al-Rawi, A. Khadouri, and A. W. Al-Mufti. 1976. Indirect sources of mercury poisoning in the Iraqi epidemic. *Bull World Health Organization* 53(Suppl.): 129–32.

Bakir, F., S. F. Damluji, L. Amin-Zaki, M. Murtadha, A. Khalidi, N. Y. Al-Rawi, S. Tikriti, H. I. Dhahir, T. W. Clarkson, J. C. Smith, and R. A. Doherty. 1973. Methylmercury poisoning in Iraq. *Science* 181: 230–40.

Bakir, F., S. Tikriti, H. Rustam, S. F. Al-Damluji, and H. Shahristani. 1980. Clinical and epidemiological aspects of methylmercury poisoning. *Postgraduate Med J* 56: 1–10.

Barker, M. H., H. A. Lindberg, and M. E. Thomas. 1942. Sudden death and mercurial diuretics. *JAMA* 119(13): 1001–4.

Bassler, A. 1935. An abortive and curative treatment for common colds. *Laryngoscope* 45: 877–85.

Bedoya, M. 2001. Gold Mining and Indigenous Conflict in Peru: Lessons from the

Amarakaeri. Project counseling services (PCS), Peru, 2001. www.undp.org/cso/resource/CSO_perspectives/beyondSG/chapter8.pdf.

Bernier, J., P. Brousseau, K. Krystyniak, H. Tryphonas, and M. Fournier. 1995. Immunotoxicity of heavy metals in relation to Great Lakes. *Environ Health Perspect* 103(Suppl. 9): 23–34.

Beuter, A., and R. Edwards. 2004. Effect of chronic exposure to methylmercury on eye movements in Cree subjects. *Int Arch Occup Environ Health* 77(2): 97–107.

Bigazzi, P. E. 1994. Autoimmunity and heavy metals. *Lupus* 3: 449–53.

Bornhausen, M., H. R. Müsch, and H. Greim. 1980. Operant behavior performance changes in rats after prenatal methylmercury exposure. *Toxicology and Applied Pharmacology* 56: 305–10.

Bovet, P., F. Perret, C. Shamlaye, R. Darioli, and F. Paccaud. 1997. The Seychelles heart study II: Methods and basic findings. *Seychelles Medical and Dental Journal.* www.seychelles.net/smdj/97issue/orig2.htm.

Brewer, J. H. 1939. The antibacterial effects of the organic mercurial compounds. *JAMA* 112(20): 2009–18.

Brieger, G. H. 1967. Therapeutic conflicts and the American medical profession in the 1860's. *Bull Hist Med* 41(3): 215–22.

Brown, G., L. Freidfeld, M. Kissin, W. Modell, and R. Sussman. 1942. Deaths immediately following the intravenous administration of mercupurin. *JAMA* 119(13): 1004–5.

Buckley, M. S., A. D. Goff, W. E. Knapp. 2004. Fish oil interaction with warfarin. *Ann Pharmacother* 38(1): 50–52.

Budtz-Jørgensen, E., P. Grandjean, and P. Weihe. 2007. Separation of risks and benefits of seafood intake. *Environ Health Perspect* 115: 323–27.

Burger, J., and M. Gochfeld. 2004. Mercury in canned tuna: White versus light and temporal variation. *Environ Res* 96(3): 239–49.

———. 2005. Heavy metals in commercial fish in New Jersey. *Environ Health Perspect* 99: 403–12.

———. 2006. Mercury in fish available in supermarkets in Illinois: Are there regional differences? *Sci Total Environ* 367: 1010–16.

Burros, M. 2001. Problematic partnership: Heart Association's certifications undermine charity's credibility, critics say. *New York Times.* November 6. http://no-smoking.org/nov97/11-06-1.html.

California Department of Justice. 2003. Attorney General Lockyer pushes grocers to warn consumers about mercury in fish. Press release, Office of the Attorney General, January 17. http://ag.ca.gov/newsalerts/release.php?id=764.

Canadian Press. 1979. St. Clair commercial fishing to resume after 9-year ban. November 3.

Cargill. 2004. History. www.cargill.com/about/history/history.htm.

Cargill Switzerland. 2004. www.cargill.com/worldwide/switzerland.htm.

CBC Digital Archives. 1970. "The 'water's no good.'" November 1. http:// archives.cbc.ca/IDC-1-70-1178-6450/disasters_tragedies/grassy_Narrows _mercury_Pollution/clip1.

———. 1974. A clear and present danger. November 6. http://archives.cbc. ca/400d.asp?id=1-70-1178-6459.

———. 1974. Mercury rising: The poisoning of Grassy Narrows. November 7. http://archives.cbc.ca/500f.asp?id=1-70-1178-6612.

———. 1975. "Are Indians slowly dying?" August 20. http://Archives.cbc.ca/ 400d.asp?id=1-70-1178-6455.

———. 1975. Grassy Narrows disaster. September 23. http://archives.cbc.ca/ 500f.asp?id=1-70-1178-6465.

———. 1975. Ontario admits: "We Have a Problem." September 29. http:// archives.cbc.ca/400d.asp?id=1-70-1178-6458.

———. 1976. Fishing for fun and death. March 23. http://archives.cbc.ca/ 400d.asp?id=1-70-1178-6460.

———. 1976. Lessons in genocide. January 14. http://archives.cbc.ca/ 500f.asp?id=1-70-1178-6466.

———. 1983. Community in crisis. March 15. http://archives.cbc.ca/ 400d.asp?id=1-70-1178-6457.

———. 1985. Compensation and shame. *CBC News Toronto*. November 25. http://archives.cbc.ca/400d.asp?id=1-70-1178-6456.

CDC. 2001. Blood and hair mercury levels in young children and women of childbearing age—United States, 1999. *MMWR* 50(8): 140–43. 2 March.

———. 2004. Blood mercury levels in young children and childbearing-aged women—United States, 1999–2002. *MMWR* 53(43): 1018–20. www.cdc .gov/mmwr/preview/mmwrhtml/mm5343a5.htm.

———. 2008. Heart disease. www.cdc.gov/HeartDisease/index.htm.

Chicken of the Sea. 2008. Our company. www.chickenofthesea.com/ history.aspx.

Chicourel, E., A. M. Sakuma, O. Zenebon, and A. Tenuta-Filho. 2001. Ineffi-cacy of cooking methods on mercury reduction from shark. *Arch Lat Am Nutr* 51(3): 288–92.

Children's Health and the Environment in the Faroes. 2004. About the Faroes. www.chef-project.dk/aboutthefaroes.html.

Choy, C. M., C. W. Lam, L. T. Cheung, C. M. Briton-Jones, L. P. Cheung, and C. J. Haines. 2002. Infertility, blood mercury concentrations and dietary seafood consumption: A case-control study. *BJOG* 109(10): 1121–25.

Clarkson, T. W. 1976. Exposure to methylmercury in Grassy Narrows and

White Dog Reserves: An interim report. Ottawa Health and Welfare Canada.

————. 1993. Mercury: Major issues in environmental health. *Environ Health Perspect* 100: 31–38.

————. 1997. The toxicology of mercury. *Crit Rev Clin Lab Sci* 34(4): 360–403.

Clarkson, T., C. Cox, P. W. Davidson, and G. Myers. 1998. Mercury in fish. *Science*. 279: 459–60.

Clarkson, T. W., L. Magos, C. Cox, M. R. Greenwood, L. Amin-Zaki, M. A. Majeed, and S. F. Al-Damluji. 1981. Tests of efficacy of antidotes for removal of methylmercury in human poisoning during the Iraq outbreak. *J Pharm and Exp Thera* 218(1): 74–83.

Clarkson, T., L. Magos, and G. Myers. 2003. The toxicology of mercury: Current exposures and clinical manifestations. *N Engl J Med* 349: 1731–37.

Clarkson, T. W., and R. E. Shapiro. 1971. The absorption of mercury from food: Its significance and new methods of removing mercury from the body. In: *Mercury in Man's Environment: Proceedings of a Symposium*, Royal Society of Canada, February 15–16, 1971, p. 124.

Clarkson, T. W., H. Small, and T. Norseth. 1971. The effect of a thiol containing resin on the gastrointestinal and fecal excretion of methylmercury compounds in experimental animals. Federation proceedings. Abstracts, 55th annual meeting, Chicago, IL, April 12–17, 1971. *Federation of American Societies for Experimental Biology* 30(2).

————. 1973. Excretion and absorption of methylmercury after polythiol resin treatment. *Arch Environ Health* 26: 173–76.

Clarkson, T. W., J. J. Strain, and M. C. Archer. 2000. Nutrition-toxicology: Evolutionary aspects—Introduction. *Eur J Nutr* 39: 49–52.

Clendening, L. 1942. *Sourcebook of Medical History*. New York: Dover, p. 119.

Clinton, B. 2004. *My Life*. New York: Knopf.

Clinton, H. 2003. *Living History*. New York: Simon and Schuster.

CMA. 2003. Resolution 516, introduced by the California delegation: Mercury in food as a human health hazard. Reference Committee E. May 5.

Columbus, C. 1490s. A letter to the king and queen of Spain. University of Oklahoma College of Law Center. www.law.ou.edu/hist/columlet.html.

Committee Minutes. 1951. Hat makers and hat finishers locals no. 10 and 11. One-Hundredth Anniversary Celebration, Hotel Green, Danbury, CT, May 5.

Corish, J. L., ed. 1927. *Health Knowledge*. New York: Medical Book Distributors, p. 1149.

Coughlin, C. 2002. *Saddam: King of Terror*. New York: HarperCollins.

Covington, M. B. 2004. Omega-3 fatty acids. *American Family Physician* 70(1): 133–40.

Cox, C., D. Marsh, G. Myers, and T. Clarkson. 1995. Analysis of data on delayed development from the 1971–72 outbreak of methylmercury poisoning in Iraq: Assessment of influential points. *Neurotoxicology* 16(4): 727–30.

Creber, C., and T. Bharwada. 2003. Dow to begin phase 2 of St. Clair River sediment removal project in May. *Dow Manufacturing News* (Sarnia, ON, Canada), April 25. www.dow.com/dow_news/manufacturing/2003/20030425a.htm.

Crook, F. 1971. Rare happening before U.S. Supreme Court: Canadians to argue the case for DOW. *Globe and Mail*, January 11.

Crump, K. S., C. Van Landingham, C. Shamlaye, C. Cox, P. W. Davidson, G. J. Myers, and T. W. Clarkson. 2000. Benchmark concentrations for methylmercury obtained from the Seychelles Child Development Study. *Environ Health Perspect* 108(3): 257–63.

Curtis, P. 2003. Iraq's scientists get a new academy. *Guardian*, November 27. www.ocupationwatch.org/article.php?id-1989.

Dahan, S. S., and H. Orfaly. 1964. Electrocardiographic changes in mercury poisoning. *Am J Cardiology* 14: 178–83.

Daley, C. A., K. Harrison, P. Doyle, A. Abbott, G. Nader, and S. Larson. 2005. Effect of feeding practices on phytoestrogen, omega-3, conjugated linoleic acid and total fatty acid composition in red meat. October 31. http://ari.calstate.edu/research/pdf/03-5-045/FinalReport-03-5-045.pdf.

Damluji, S. 1962. Mercurial poisoning with the fungicide Granosan M. *J Fac Med Baghdad* 4: 83–103.

Damluji, S. F., L. Amin-Zaki, and S. B. Elhassani. 1972. Mercury in the environment. *Brit Med J* 4: 489.

Damluji, S., and S. Tikriti. 1972. Mercury poisoning from wheat. *Brit Med J* 1: 804.

Darden, T. F. 1951. *Historical Sketch of the Naval Administration of the Government of American Samoa, April 17, 1900–July 1, 1951*. Washington, DC: U.S. Government Printing Office and Naval Department.

Davidson, P. W. 2003. Methylmercury: A story of loaves and fishes. In: *Pollution, Toxic Chemicals, and Mental Retardation: A National Summit.* American Association on Mental Retardation, Racine, WI, July 22–24, 2003. www.aamr.org/ToxicsandMentalRetardation/pdf/web_paper_5_Davidson.pdf.

Davidson, P. W., D. Palumbo, G. J. Myers, C. Cox, C. F. Shamlaye, J. Sloan-Reeves, E. Cernichiari, G. E. Wilding, and T. W. Clarkson. 2000. Neurodevelopmental outcomes of Seychellois children from the pilot cohort at 108 months following prenatal exposure to methylmercury from maternal fish diet. *Environ Res* 84(Section A): 1–11.

Davies, R., and G. Davies. 1996. A comparative chronology of money: Monetary history from ancient times to the present day, 1500–1599. Based on Davies, G., *A History of Money from Ancient Times to the Present Day*, rev. ed. (Cardiff: University of Wales Press, 1996, p. 716). www.ex.ac .uk/~Rdavies/arian/amser/chrono6.html.

Debes, F., E. Budtz-Jørgensen, P. Weihe, R. F. White, and P. Grandjean. 2006. Impact of prenatal methylmercury exposure on neurobehavioral function at age 14 years. *Neurotoxicol Teratol* 28(5): 536–47.

De Forest, C. 1944. Reminiscing in the attic of the Lane Medical Library: Organization and early work at Lane Hospital. *Stanford Med Bull* 2(1): 15–19.

———. 1949. Recollections of the Lane Hospital operating room: 1900 to 1903. *Stanford Med Bull* 7(3): 112–14 and IIJ.

DeGraff, A. C., and R. A. Lehman. 1942. The acute toxicity of mercurial diuretics. *JAMA* 119(13): 998–1001.

DeGraff, A. C., and J. E. Nadler. 1942. A review of the toxic manifestations of mercurial diuretics in man. *JAMA* 119(13): 1006–11.

Dickman, M. D., and K. M. C. Leung. 1998. Mercury and organochlorine exposure from fish consumption in Hong Kong. *Chemosphere* 37(5): 991–1015.

Dinehart, S. M., R. Dillard, S. S. Raimer, S. Diven, R. Cobos, and R. Pupo. 1988. Cutaneous manifestations of acrodynia (pink disease). *Arch Dermatol* 124: 107–9.

D'Itri, P., and F. D'Itri. 1977. *Mercury Contamination: A Human Tragedy*. New York: Wiley.

Dow Chemical. 2004. Company profile. www.stanford.edu/group/SICD/ DowChemical/dow.html.

Dye, B. A., S. E. Schober, C. F. Dillon, R. L. Jones, C. Fryar, M. McDowell, and T. H. Sinks. 2005. Urinary mercury concentrations associated with dental restorations in adult women aged 16–49 years: United States, 1999–2000. *Occ Environ Med* 62: 368–75.

Egeland, G. M., and J. P. Middaugh. 1997. Balancing fish consumption benefits with mercury exposure. *Science* 278: 1904–5.

Ekino, S., M. Susa, T. Ninomiya, K. Imamura, and T. Kitamura. 2007. Minamata disease revisited: An update on the acute and chronic manifestations of methylmercury poisoning. *J Neurol Sci* 262(1–2): 131–44.

Ekstrom, E. B., E. G. Malcolm, J. K. Schaefer, and F. M. Morel. 2006. Possible biotic and abiotic sources of methylmercury in the ocean. Poster presentation for Mercury 2006: 8th International Conference on Mercury as

a Global Pollutant, Madison, WI, August 6–11, 2006. www.mercury2006
.org/.

Environment Canada. 2007. Canadian Remedial Action Plans: St. Clair
River Area of Concern. www.ec.gc.ca/raps-pas/default.asp?lang=En&n=
A2A5595F-1.

Evers, D. C., Y. J. Han, C. T. Driscoll, N. C. Kamman, M. W. Goodale, K. F.
Lambert, T. M. Holsen, C. Y. Chen, T. A. Clair, and T. Butler. 2007. Biological mercury hotspots in the northeastern United States and southeast-
ern Canada. *BioScience* 57(1): 29–43.

Faleomavaega, E. F. H. 2002. Del Monte and Heinz request meeting with Faleomavaega to discuss future status of StarKist. Press release. Washington,
DC: U.S. House of Representatives, June 13. www.house.gov/list/press/as00
_faleomavaega/starkistmeetfaleomavaega.html.

———. 2003. Faleomavaega protects American Samoa's tuna industry
from Micronesian competition. Press release. Washington, DC: U.S.
House of Representatives, June 19. www.house.gov/apps/list/press/as00
_faleomavaega/eniprotectstuna.html.

———. 2003. Statement of the Honorable Eni F. H. Faleomavaega, before
Special Industry Committee no. 25, U.S. Department of Labor Wage and
Hour Division, regarding the minimum wage in American Samoa.
Fagatogo, Samoa, June 16. www.house.gov/faleomavaega/speech-030616
-minimumwage.htm.

———. 2003. Tangled nets and heaps of stones: The future of the tuna canneries in American Samoa. *Pacific Magazine.* May. www.pacificmagazine
.net/pm52003/pmdefault.php?urlarticleid=0012.

Falk, C. R., and S. P. Aplington. 1936. Studies on the bactericidal action of
phenol and Merthiolate used alone and in mixtures. *Am J Hyg* 24:
285–308.

Feinstein, D. 2000. Letter to Ms. Diane E. Thompson, September 27.
www.cfsan.fda.gov/~acrobat/hgcong73.pdf.

Fialka, J. 2003. EPA and FDA, long in dispute. *Wall Street Journal,* October
21, A1.

"The Fish Risk," *20/20,* January 12, 2001.

Fishinfo. 2006. Living off the sea in the Faroes Islands. www.fishin
.fo/get.asp?gid=dC2FA95B7-E790-4B96-9CAF-FA37E6F236D1Living
off the sea.

Fitzgerald, W. F., and T. W. Clarkson. 1991. Mercury and monomethyl-
mercury: Present and future concerns. *Environ Health Perspect* 96:
159–66.

Flannery, M. A. 2004. *Civil War Pharmacy: A History of Drugs, Drug Supply and Provision, and Therapeutics for the Union and Confederacy*. New York: Hawthorn Press.

From dropout to dictator. 2003. *Sunday Times* South Africa. March 23. www.suntimes.co.za/2003/03/23/insight/in01.asp.

Frustaci, A., N. Magnavita, C. Chimenti, M. Caldarulo, E. Sabbioni, R. Pietra, et al. 1999. Marked elevation of myocardial trace elements in idiopathic dilated cardiomyopathy compared with secondary cardiac dysfunction. *J Am Coll Cardiol* 33(6): 1578–83.

Fukuda, Y., K. Ushijima, T. Kitano, M. Sakamoto, and M. Futatsuka. 1999. An analysis of subjective complaints in a population living in a methyl-mercury-polluted area. *Environ Res* 81(Section A): 100–107.

Futatsuka, M., T. Kitano, M. Shono, M. Nagano, J. Wakamiya, K. Miyamoto, K. Ushijima, T. Inaoka, Y. Fukuda, M. Nakagawa, K. Arimura, and M. Osame. 2005. Long-term follow-up study of health status in population living in methylmercury-polluted area. *Environ Sci* (December): 239–82.

Garrison, F. H. 1929. *An Introduction to the History of Medicine*. Philadelphia: W.B. Saunders, pp. 136, 191, 219, 241, 285.

Geier, D. A., and M. R. Geier. 2006. A meta-analysis epidemiological assess-ment of neurodevelopmental disorders following vaccines administered from 1994 through 2000 in the United States. *Neuro Endocrinol Lett* 27(4): 410–13.

Geier, M. R., and D. A. Geier. 2003. Neurodevelopmental disorders after thimerosal-containing vaccines: A brief communication. *Exp Biol Med* 228: 660–64.

———. 2003. Thimerosal in childhood vaccines, neurodevelopmental disor-ders, and heart disease in the United States. *J Am Phys Surg* 8(1): 6–11.

Giles, J. 2003. Iraqis draw up blueprint for revitalizing science academy. *Nature*. 426 (December): 484.

Gillet, R., M. A. McCoy, and D. G. Itano. 2004. Status of the United States western Pacific tuna purse seine fleet and factors affecting its future. SOEST 02-01. JIMAR contribution 02-344. www.SOEST.Hawaii.edu/PFRP/pdf/gpa_amer_samoa.pdf.

Goldwater, L. 1972. *A History of Quicksilver*. Baltimore: York Press.

Graham, P. 2003. Quiet loner gained respect through killing: Saddam Hus-sein: Portrait of a dictator. *National Post*, January 11, A1.

Grandjean, P., K. Murata, E. Budtz-Jørgensen, and P. Weihe. 2004. Cardiac autonomic activity in methylmercury neurotoxicity: 14-year follow-up of a Faroese birth cohort. *J Pediatr* 144: 169–76.

Grandjean, P., P. Weihe, and J. B. Nielsen. 1994. Methylmercury: Significance of intrauterine and postnatal exposures. *Clin Chem* 40(7): 1395–1400.

Grandjean, P., P. Weihe, R. F. White, and F. Debes. 1998. Cognitive performance of children prenatally exposed to "safe" levels of methylmercury. *Environ Res* 77(Section A): 165–72.

Grandjean, P., R. F. White, A. Nielsen, D. Cleary, and E. C. de Oliveira Santos. 1999. Methylmercury neurotoxicity in Amazonian children downstream from gold mining. *Environ Health Perspect* 107(7): 587–91.

Greiner, T., and H. Gold. 1953. Method for therapeutic evaluation of diuretic
agents administered orally. *JAMA* 152(12): 1130–31.

Grun, B. 1982. *The Timetables of History*. New York: Simon and Schuster, p. 5.

Guallar, E., I. Sanz-Gallardo, P. Van't Veer, P. Bode, A. Aro, J. Gomez-Aracena,
et al. 2002. Mercury, fish oils, and the risk of myocardial infarction. *N Eng
J Med* 347(22): 1747–54.

Guy, R. A. 1923. The history of cod liver oil as a remedy. *Am J Dis Child* 26:
112–16.

Haggerty, R. F., T. B. Calhoon, W. H. Lee, and J. T. Cuttino. 1960. Human
cartilage grafts stored in Merthiolate. *Surg Gyn Obst* (February): 229–33.

Hamilton, N. 2003. *Bill Clinton: An American Journey, Great Expectations*.
New York: Random House.

Haq, I. U. L. 1963. Agrosan poisoning in man. *Brit Med J* 1: 1579–82.

Harada, M. 1978. Congenital Minamata disease: Intrauterine methylmercury
poisoning. *Teratology* 18: 285–88.

———. 1995. Minamata disease: Methylmercury poisoning in Japan caused
by environmental pollution. *Critical Reviews in Toxicology* 25(1): 1–24.

Harada, M., T. Fujino, T. Akagi, and S. Nishigaki. 1976. Epidemiological and
clinical study and historical background of mercury pollution on Indian
reservations in northwestern Ontario, Canada. *Bull Inst Constit Med*
26(3–4): 169–84.

Harada, M., T. Fujino, T. Oorui, S. Nakachi, T. Nou, T. Kizaki, Y. Hitomi, N.
Nakano, N., and H. Ohno. 2005. Follow-up study of mercury pollution in
indigenous tribe reservations in the province of Ontario, Canada,
1975–2002. *Bull Environ Contam Toxicol* 74: 689–97.

Hechtman, K. 2003. Clearcut defiance: The Ojibway of Grassy Narrows,
Ontario, stand up to Montreal-based pulp and paper monolith Abitibi-
Consolidated. *Montreal Mirror*. www.montrealmirror.com/ARCHIVES/
2003/032003/news3.html.

Heilmann, C., P. Grandjean, P. Weihe, F. Nielsen, and E. Budtz-Jørgensen.
2006. Reduced antibody responses to vaccinations in children exposed to
polychlorinated biphenyls. *PLoS Med* 3(8): 1352–59. www.plosmedicine
.org.

Heinz. 2004. Heinz Milestones. www.heinz.com/jsp/milestones.jsp.

Hightower, J. M. 2001. The danger of mercury poisoning from fish. *San Francisco Medicine* 74(3, March).

———. 2002. Letter to Senator Dianne Feinstein, November 20.

Hightower, J. M., and J. Mates. 2003. Mercury in food as a human health hazard. Resolution 112-03, endorsed by the San Francisco Medical Society, Reference Committee A, March 22–25.

Hightower, J. M., and D. Moore. 2003. Mercury levels in high-end consumers of fish. *Environ Health Perspect* 111(4): 604–8.

Hightower, J. M., A. O'Hare, and G. T. Hernandez. 2006. Blood mercury reporting in NHANES: Identifying Asian, Pacific Islander, Native American and multiracial groups. *Environ Health Perspect* 114(2): 173–75.

Hirschhorn, N., R. G. Feldman, and I. A. Greaves. 2001. Abraham Lincoln's little blue pills. *Perspectives in Biology and Medicine* 44(3): 315–32.

Hites, R. A., J. A. Foran, D. O. Carpenter, M. C. Hamilton, B. A. Knuth, and S. J. Schwager. 2004. Global assessment of organic contaminants in farmed salmon. *Science* 203: 226–29.

Howard, Marion E., ed. 1952. *Modern Drug Encyclopedia and Therapeutic Index*, 5th ed. New York: Drug Publications.

Hughes, E. 1973. Pink Death in Iraq. *Reader's Digest* 103:134–138. November.

———. 1973. How the Pink Death Came to Iraq. *London Sunday Times*, September 9.

Hyson, J. M. 2006. Amalgam: Its history and perils. *CDA Journal* 34(3): 215–29.

IDDRA (UK) Ltd. 2004. Analysis of the impact on ACP countries of opening up the EU import market for canned tuna. Executive summary. Commissioned by CTA and the commonwealth secretariat. February. http://agritrade.cta.int/tuna_study_30pager_EN.pdf.

Igata, A. 1993. Epidemiological and congenital features of Minamata disease. *Environ Res* 63: 157–69.

Indian and Northern Affairs Canada. 2004. English-Wabigoon River mercury compensation. April 23. www.ainc-inac.gc.ca/pr/info/ewr_e.html.

International Joint Commission. 2007. About the Great Lakes Water Quality Agreement. November 22, 1978. www.ijc.org/rel/agree/quality.html.

International Trade Centre. 1999. Sub Regional Trade Expansion in Southern Africa: Supply Survey on Seychelles' Fish and Fish Products. July–August. www.intracen.org/sstp/Survey/fish/fishsey.html.

Jacobs, M. N., A. Covaci, and P. Schepens. 2002. Investigation of selected persistent organic pollutants in farmed Atlantic salmon (*Salmo salar*), salmon aquaculture feed, and fish oil components of the feed. *Environ Sci Technol* 36: 2797–2805.

Jamieson, W. A., and H. M. Powell. 1931. Merthiolate as a preservative for biological products. *Am J Hyg* 14: 218–24.

Japan Times. 2004. Top court holds state to account for Minamata. http://search.japantimes.co.jp/cgi-bin/nn20041016a2.html. 16 October.

JIFSAN. The Joint Institute for Food Safety and Applied Nutrition Annual Report 1998–1999. http://web.archive.org/web/20020616124945 or http://www.jifsan.umd.edu/Rev99AnRep.htm.

Karsh, E., and I. Rautsi. 1991. *Saddam Hussein: A Political Biography*. New York: Free Press.

Keating, M. H. 1997. *Mercury Study Report to Congress*. Vol. 2, *An Inventory of Anthropogenic Mercury Emissions in the United States*. U.S. Environmental Protection Agency. December. www.epa.gov/ttn/oarpg/t3/reports/volume2.pdf.

Knobeloch, L. M., M. Ziarnick, H. A. Anderson, and V. N. Dodson. 1995. Imported seabass as a source of mercury exposure: A Wisconsin case study. *Environ Health Perspect* 103(6): 604–6.

Korns, R. F. 1972. The frustrations of Bettye Russow. *Nutrition Today* (December): 21–23.

Kraepiel, A. M. I., K. Keller, H. B. Chin, E. G. Malcolm, and F. M. M. Morel. 2003. Sources and variations of mercury in tuna. *Environ Sci Technol* 37: 5551–58.

Kris-Etherton, P. M., W. S. Harris, and L. J. Appel. 2002. Fish consumption, fish oil, omega-3 fatty acids, and cardiovascular disease. *Circulation* 106: 2747–57.

Kunin, R. A. 1989. Snake oil. *West J Med* 151(2): 208.

LeBlanc, T. J., and M. B. Welborn. 1936. The common cold: The effect of Merthiolate as a therapeutic agent. *Am J Hyg* 24: 343–49.

Leung, T. Y., C. M. Choy, S. F. Yim, C. W. Lam, and C. J. Haines. 2001. Whole blood mercury concentrations in sub-fertile men in Hong Kong. *Aust N Z J Obstet Gynaecol* 41(1): 75–77.

Lewis, L. R. 1997. Peru, Coca trade, and environment. Case number 437. *Trade and Environment* database. http://gurukul.ucc.american.edu/ted/perucoca.htm. 29 May.

Luke, A. F. 2006. Science shows WIC moms and children will reap health benefits from more canned tuna. U.S. Tuna Foundation press release, August 4. www.tunafoundation.org/mediacenter/2006_releases/08_04_06.html.

Mackenzie, C. A., A. Lockridge, and M. Keith. 2005. Declining sex ratio in a first nation community. *Environ Health Perspect* 113(10): 1295–98.

Mackey, S. 2002. *The Reckoning: Iraq and the Legacy of Saddam Hussein*. New York: W.W. Norton.

Mahaffey, K. R. 2004. Fish and shellfish as dietary sources of methylmercury and the omega-3 fatty acids, eicosahexaenoic acid and docosahexaenoic acid: Risks and benefits. *Environ Res* 95(3): 414–28.

———. 2005. Mercury exposure: Medical and public health issues. *Trans Am Clin Climatol Assoc* 116: 127–54.

Mahaffey, K. R., and G. E. Rice. 1997. *Mercury Study Report to Congress.* Vol. 4, *An Assessment of Exposure to Mercury in the United States.* U.S. Environmental Protection Agency, Office of Air Quality Planning and Standards. December. www.epa.gov/ttn/oarpg/t3/reports/volume4.pdf.

Marcus, J. 1938. *The Jew in the Medieval World: A Sourcebook, 315–1791.* New York: JPS, pp. 51–55. Also available as "Jewish History Sourcebook: The Expulsion from Spain, 1492 CE," www.fordham.edu/halsall/jewish/1492-jews-spain1.html.

Marine Fisheries Review. 1989. Salmon culture in the Faroe Islands—Faeroe Islands—Foreign Fishery Developments. Fall. www.findarticles.com/p/articles/mi_m3089/is_n4_v51/ai_9346480.

Marsh, D. O., T. W. Clarkson, C. Cox, G. J. Myers, L. Amin-Zaki, and S. Tikriti. 1987. Fetal methylmercury poisoning: Relationship between concentration in single strands of maternal hair and child effects. *Arch neurol* 44: 1017–22.

Marsh, D. O., T. W. Clarkson, G. J. Myers, P. W. Davidson, C. Cox, E. Cernichiari, M. A. Tanner, W. Lednar, C. Shamlaye, O. Choisy, C. Hoareau, and M. Berlin. 1995. The Seychelles study of fetal methylmercury exposure and child development: Introduction. *Neurotoxicology* 16(4): 583–96.

Marsh, D. O., G. J. Myers, T. W. Clarkson, L. Amin-Zaki, S. Tikriti, and M. A. Majeed. 1980. Fetal methylmercury poisoning: Clinical and toxicological data on 29 cases. *Ann Neurol* 7(4): 348–53.

Marsh, D. O., M. D. Turner, J. C. Smith, P. Allen, and N. Richdale. 1995. Fetal methylmercury study in a Peruvian fish-eating population. *Neurotoxicology* 16(4): 171–726.

Marsh, D. O., M. Turner, J. C. Smith, W. J. Choi, and T. W. Clarkson. 1974. Methylmercury in human populations eating large quantities of marine fish. II. American Samoa: Cannery workers and fishermen. *Proc. First International Mercury Conference, Barcelona,* vol. 2, pp. 235–39. Fabrica National de Moneda y Timbre. May.

Matthews, A. D. 1983. Mercury content of commercially important fish of the Seychelles, and hair mercury levels of a selected part of the population. *Environ Res* 30(2): 305–12.

McClaskey, E. M., and E. L. Michalets. 2007. Subdural hematoma after a fall in an elderly patient taking high-dose omega-3 fatty acids with warfarin and aspirin: Case report and review of the literature. *Pharmacotherapy* 27(1): 152–60.

Mercury in the environment. Editorial. 1972. *Br Med J* 2: 605–6.

Mercury 2006: 8th International Conference on Mercury as a Global Pollutant. Madison, WI, August 6–11. www.mercury2006.org/.

Mergler, D., S. Belanger, F. Larribe, M. Panisset, R. Bowler, M. Baldwin, J. Lebel, and K. Hudnell. 1998. Preliminary evidence of neurotoxicity associated with eating fish from the upper St. Lawrence River Lakes. *Neurotoxicology* 19(4–5): 691–702.

Mezei, E. *Tooth Traitors*. 1990. www.talkinternational.com/PDF/tooth_traitors.pdf#search=%22Tooth%20Traitors%22.

Miljøministeriet. 2003. AMAP Greenland and the Faroe Islands 1997–2001. Faroe Islands: Sociocultural environment, lifestyle, health and contaminant exposure. http://www2.mst.dk/common/Udgivramme/Frame.asp?pg =http://www2.mst.dk/udgiv/Publications/2003/87-7972-477- 9/html/kap06_eng.htm.

Miller, J., and L. Mylroie. 1990. *Saddam Hussein and the Crisis in the Gulf*. New York: Random House.

Morgan, J. N., M. R. Berry, and R. L. Graves. 1997. Effects of commonly used cooking practices on total mercury concentration in fish and their impact on exposure assessments. *J Expo Anal Environ Epidemiol* 7(1): 19–33.

Morrissey, M. T. 2004. Mercury content in Pacific troll-caught albacore tuna. *J Aquatic Food Product Technology* 13(4): 41.

Mortensen, J. D., L. A. Weed, and J. H. Grindlay. 1954. Maintaining sterility during storage of arterial homographs. *J Lab Clin Med* 44(4): 604–8.

Morton, H. E., L. E. North, and F. B. Engley. 1948. The bacteriostatic and bactericidal actions of some mercurial compounds on hemolytic streptococci. *JAMA* 136(1): 37–41.

Mozaffarian, D., and E. B. Rimm. 2006. Fish intake, contaminants, and human health: Evaluating the risks and the benefits. *JAMA* 296(15): 1885–99.

Munthe, T., ed. 2002. *The Saddam Hussein Reader*. New York: Thunder Mountain Press.

Murata, K., P. Weihe, E. Budtz-Jørgensen, P. J. Jørgensen, and P. Grandjean. 2004. Delayed brainstem auditory evoked potential latencies in 14-year-old children exposed to methylmercury. *J Pediatr* 144: 177–83.

Murphy, S. C., L. J. Whited, L. C. Rosenberry, B. H. Hammond, D. K. Bandler, and K. J. Boor. 2001. Fluid milk vitamin fortification compliance in New York State. *J Dairy Sci* 84: 2813–20.

Myers, G. J., P. W. Davidson, C. Cox, C. Shamlaye, E. Cernichiari, and T. W. Clarkson. 2000. Twenty-seven years studying the human neurotoxicity of methylmercury exposure. *Environ Res*, Section A (83): 275–85.

Myers, G. J., P. W. Davidson, C. Cox, C. F. Shamlaye, D. Palumbo,

E. Cernichiari, J. Sloane-Reeves, G. E. Wilding, J. Kost, Li-Shan Huang, and T. W. Clarkson. 2003. Prenatal methylmercury exposure from ocean fish consumption in the Seychelles Child Development Study. *Lancet*. 36: 1686–92.

Myers, G. J., P. W. Davidson, C. F. Shamlaye, C. D. Axtell, E. Cernichiari, O. Choisy, A. Choi, C. Cox, and T. Clarkson. 1997. Effects of prenatal methylmercury exposure from a high fish diet on developmental milestones in the Seychelles child development study. *Neurotoxicology* 18(3): 819–30.

Myers, G. J., D. O. Marsh, C. Cox, P. W. Davidson, C. F. Shamlaye, M. A. Tanner, A. Choi, E. Cernichiari, O. Choisy, and T. W. Clarkson. 1995. A pilot neurodevelopmental study of Seychellois children following in utero exposure to methylmercury from a maternal fish diet. *Neurotoxicology* 16(4): 629–38.

Myers, G. J., D. O. Marsh, P. W. Davidson, C. Cox, C. F. Shamlaye, M. Tanner, A. Choi, E. Cernichiari, O. Choisy, and T. W. Clarkson. 1995. Main neurodevelopmental study of Seychellois children following in utero exposure to methylmercury from a maternal fish diet: Outcome at six months. *Neurotoxicology* 16(4): 653–64.

National Academy of Sciences. 2000. *Toxicological Effects of Methylmercury*. Washington, DC: Author. July. http://nap.edu/books/0309071402/html.

National Center for Health Statistics. 2005. NHANES 1999–2000 and NHANES 2001–2002 Public use data files. www.cdc.gov/nchs/about/major/nhanes/NHANES99_00.htm. And www.cdc.gov/nchs/about/major/nhanes/nhanes01-02.htm.

Neal, P. A., R. H. Flinn, T. I. Edwards, et al. 1941. Mercurialism and its control in the felt hat industry. Federal Security Agency, U.S. Public Health Service. Public Health Bulletin no. 263.

Neal, P. A., R. R. Jones, J. J. Bloomfield, J. M. Dalla Valle, and T. I. Edwards. 1937. A study of chronic mercurialism in the hatters' fur-cutting industry. *Public Health Bulletin no. 234*. U.S. Treasury Department, Public Health Service.

Nesheim, Malden C., and A. L. Yaktine, eds. 2006. *Seafood Choices: Balancing Benefits and Risks*. Committee on Nutrient Relationships in Seafood: Selections to Balance Benefits and Risks, Food and Nutrition Board. Washington, DC: National Academies Press. October.

Newschaffer, C. J., L. A. Croen, J. Daniels, E. Giarelli, J. K. Grether, S. E. Levy, D. S. Mandell, L. A. Miller, J. Pinto-Martin, J. Reaven, A. M. Reynolds, C. E. Rice, D. Schendel, and G. C. Windham. 2007. The epidemiology of autism spectrum disorders. *Annu Rev Public Health* 28: 235–58.

Nielsen, J. B., and P. Hultman. 2002. Mercury-induced autoimmunity in mice. *Environ Health Perspect* 110(Suppl. 5): 877–81.

Nightingale, S. L. 1991. From the Food and Drug Administration. *JAMA*. 265(22): 2934.

NOAA Fisheries. 2004. Office of Science and Technology, International Science and Technology Division. *World Swordfish Fisheries*. Vol. 4, *South America*, part A. www.st.nmfs.gov/st3/vol4swordfish.html.

O'Carroll, R. E., G. Masterton, N. Dougall, K. P. Ebmeier, and G. M. Goodwin. 1995. The neuropsychiatric sequelae of mercury poisoning: The mad hatter's disease revisited. *British Journal of Psychiatry* 167: 95–98.

Ohio claims DOW, Wyandotte knowingly discharged mercury. 1971. *Globe and Mail*, January 11.

Oken, E., J. S. Radesky, R. O. Wright, D. C. Bellinger, C. J. Amarasiriwardena, K. P. Kleinman, H. Hu, and M. W. Gillman. 2008. Maternal fish intake during pregnancy, blood mercury levels, and child cognition at age 3 years in a U.S. cohort. *Am J Epidemiol* 167(10):1171–81.

Olivero, J., B. Johnson, and E. Arguello. 2002. Human exposure to mercury in San Jorge River Basin, Colombia (South America). *The Science of the Total Environment* 289: 41–47.

Omega-3 oil: Fish or pills. 2003. *Consumer Reports*. July.

Ontario Department of Health. Environmental Health Services Branch, Public Health Division. 1972. *The Public Health Significance of Methylmercury*. February 18.

Ontario Legislature. 1974. This document can be found in the Marion Lamm Collection, Harvard University Environmental Library, Cambridge, MA.

Open Secrets. 2004. George Bush top contributors. www.opensecrets .org/presidential/contrib.asp?id=N00008072&cycle=2004.

———. 2005. Coal mining: Top recipients. www.opensecrets.org/industries/ recips.asp?Ind=E1210.

———. 2005. Electric utilities: Top recipients. www.opensecrets.org/indus- tries/recips.asp?Ind=E08.

Ortiz-Roque, C., and Y. Lopez-Rivera. 2004. Mercury contamination in repro- ductive age women in a Caribbean Island: Vieques. *J Epidemiol Commu- nity Health* 58: 756–57.

People of the State of California, ex rel. Bill Lockyer, Attorney General of the state of California vs. Tri-Union Seafoods, LLC., Del Monte Corporation, Bum- ble Bee Seafoods, LLC, and does 1 through 499; Public Media Center vs. Tri-Union Seafoods, LLC, Del Monte Corporation (formerly sued as H.J. Heinz Co.), Bumble Bee Seafoods, LLC (formerly sued as Bumble Bee Seafoods, Inc.), and does 1 through 499. Consolidated case nos.: CGC-01-

402975-04-432394. Superior Court of California, County of San Francisco, 2006.

———. Findings of fact and conclusions of law re: preemption, MADL, and naturally occurring. April 17, 2006.

———. People's objections to court's proposed statement of decision. May 26, 2006

Pichichero, M. E. 2000. Acute otitis media: Part II. Treatment in an era of increasing antibiotic resistance. *American Family Physician* 61: 2410–16.

Pichichero, M. E., E. Cernichieri, J. Lopreiato, and J. Treanor. 2002. Mercury concentrations and metabolism in infants receiving vaccines containing thiomersal: A descriptive study. *Lancet* 360(9347): 1737–41.

Pichichero, M. E., M. B. Rennels, K. M. Edwards, M. M. Blatter, G. S. Marshall, M. Bologa, E. Wang, and E. Mills. 2005. Combined tetanus, diphtheria, and 5-component pertussis vaccine for use in adolescents and adults. *JAMA* 293(24): 3003–11.

Pichichero M. E., A. Gentile, N. Giglio, V. Umibdo, T. W. Clarkson, E. Cernichiari, G. Zareba, C. Gotelli, L. Yan, J. Treanor. 2008. Mercury levels in newborns and infants after receipt of thimerosal-containing vaccines. *Pediatrics* 121(2): 208–14.

Plaisier, M. 2000. Letter to the Honorable Dianne Feinstein from the Food and Drug Administration, December 21. www.cfsan.fda.gov/~acrobat/hgcong74.pdf.

Pombo, R., and R. Gibbons. 2005. Mercury in perspective: Fact and fiction about the debate over mercury. http://resourcescommittee.house.gov/Press/reports/mercury_in_perspective.pdf.

Poulter, G. 2007. History. The Natural Resources Institute. October 30. www.nri.org/about/history.htm.

Powell, H. M., and W. A. Jamieson. 1931. Merthiolate as a germicide. *Am J Hyg* 13: 296–310.

———. 1938. The efficiency of Merthiolate as a biological preservative after ten years' use. *Proc Indiana Acad Sci* 47(65).

Powell, H. M., W. A. Jamieson, and G. F. Kempf. 1932. The healing properties of Merthiolate. *Am J Hyg* 15: 292–97.

Prasad, V. L. 2004. Subcutaneous injection of mercury: "Warding off evil." *Environ Health Perspect* 112: 1326–28.

Puckner, W. A. 1932. Council on pharmacy and chemistry. Reports of the council. Average optimum dosage of cod liver oil. *JAMA* 98(4): 316–18.

Public Health Service. 1993. Dental Amalgam: A scientific review and recommended public health service strategy for research, education and regulation. http://web.health.gov/environment/amalgam1/ct.htm.

Purcell International. 2008. Company History. www.purcell-intl.com/history/ index.html.

Putman, J. J., and R. W. Madden. 1972. Quicksilver and slow death. *National Geographic* (October): 506–27.

Rajakumar, K. 2003. Vitamin D, cod liver oil, sunlight, and rickets: A historical perspective. *Pediatrics* 112(2): 132–35.

Ramazzini, B. 1713. *Diseases of Workers.* Reprint, Chicago: University of Chicago Press, 1983, pp. 21, 33, 53, 65.

Rhead, E. L. 1895. *Metallurgy: Extraction of silver.* London (rev. 1939), pp. 267–85. http://website.lineon.net/~petehutch/silver.pdf.

Rickey, T. 1998. Commercial fish: Eat up, despite low levels of mercury. University of Rochester. August 26. www.rochester.edu/pr/releases/med/ mercury.htm.

Riley, D. M., C. A. Newby, T. O. Leal-Almeraz, and V. M. Thomas. 2001. Assessing elemental mercury vapor exposure from cultural and religious practices. *Environ Health Perspect* 109: 779–84.

Rissanen, T., S. Voultilainen, K. Nyyssönen, T. A. Lakka, and J. T. Salonen. 2000. Fish oil-derived fatty acids, docosahexaenoic acid and docosapentanoic acid, and the risk of acute coronary events. *Circulation* 102: 2677–79.

Rosenstein, C., I. Levin, and H. Levin. 1935. The bactericidal and antiseptic action of preservatives frequently used in biological products, and the effect of these preservatives on the potencies of the products. *Am J Hyg* 21: 260–79.

Sainty, G. S. 2004. Great orders of chivalry: The military order of Santiago. www.chivalricorders.org/orders/spanish/santiago.htm.

———. 2004. Great orders of chivalry: The Spanish military orders. www.chivalricorders.org/orders/spanish/fourspan.htm.

Salonen, J. T., K. Seppänen, T. A. Lakka, R. Salonen, and G. A. Kaplan. 2000. Mercury accumulation and accelerated progression of carotid atherosclerosis: A population-based prospective 4-year follow-up study in men in eastern Finland. *Atherosclerosis* 148: 265–73.

Salonen, J. T., K. Seppänen, K. Nyyssönen, H. Korpela, J. Kauhanen, M. Kantola, et al. 1995. Intake of mercury from fish, lipid peroxidation, and the risk of myocardial infarction and coronary, cardiovascular, and any death in eastern Finish men. *Circulation* 91(3): 645–55.

Schabath, G. 2002. State to test drinking water: Dredging to clean St. Clair River at Sarnia prompts contaminant checks at 12 plants. *Detroit News,* June 3. www.mindfully.org/Water/DOW-Contaminates-Water5jun02.htm.

Scorecard. 2008. Chemical profile for methyl mercury. www.scorecard

.org/chemical-profiles/summary.tcl?edf_substance_id=22967%2d92
%2d6#ranking.

Seppanen, K., M. Kantola, R. Laatikainen, K. Nyyssonen, V. P. Valkonen, V. Kaarlopp, and J. T. Salonen. 2000. Effect of supplementation with organic selenium on mercury status as measured by mercury in pubic hair. *J Trace Elem Med Biol* 14(2): 84–87.

Sexton, A. H. 1899. *An Elemental Textbook of Metallurgy*, 2nd ed. London: Charles Griffen.

Shamlaye, C. F., D. O. Marsh, G. J. Myers, C. Cox, P. W. Davidson, O. Choisy, E. Cernichiari, A. Choi, M. A. Tanner, and T. W. Clarkson. 1995. The Seychelles Child Development Study on neurodevelopmental outcomes in children following in utero exposure to methylmercury from a maternal fish diet: Background and demographics. *Neurotoxicology* 16(4): 597–612.

Shamlaye, C., H. Shamlaye, and R. Brewer. 2004. Health in Seychelles: An overview. *Seychelles Medical and Dental Journal* 7(1): 13–20.

Sheiner, E. K., E. Sheiner, R. D. Hammel, G. Potashnik, and R. Carel. 2003. Effect of occupational exposures on male fertility: Literature review. *Ind Health* 41(2): 55–62.

Sierra Club. Clear Skies proposal weakens the Clean Air Act. www.sierra club.org/cleanair/clear_skies.asp.

Silva, I. A., J. F. Nyland, A. Gorman, A. Perisse, A. M. Ventura, E. C. O. Santos, et al. 2004. Mercury exposure, malaria, and serum antinuclear/antinucleolar antibodies in Amazon populations in Brazil: A cross sectional study. *Environmental Health* 3:11. www.ehjournal.net/content/3/1/11.

Smith, R. C., J. Spirek, J. Bratten, and D. Scott-Ireton. 1995. The Emanuel Point Ship: Archaeological investigations 1992–1995, Preliminary report. Florida Bureau of Archeological Research. www.flheritage.com/archaeology/projects/shipwrecks/emanuelpoint/stern.cfm.

Smith, W. E., and A. M. Smith. 1975. *Minamata: The Story of the Poisoning of a City, and of the People Who Choose to Carry the Burden of Courage*, 1st ed. New York: Holt, Rinehart and Winston.

Sørensen, N., K. Murata, E. Budtz-Jørgensen, P. Weihe, and P. Grandjean. 1999. Prenatal methylmercury exposure as a cardiovascular risk factor at seven years of age. *Epidemiology* 10: 370–75.

Spaeth, D. 2002. Mercury: Why the amalgam debate just won't go away. *Dental Practice Report* July–August 16–31.

Stanford University School of Medicine. 1959. *1959 Yearbook: The First Hundred Years*. Glendale, CA: Mirro-Graphic Yearbooks.

Stejskal, J., and V. D. M. Stejskal. 1999. The role of metals in autoimmunity and the link to neuroendocrinology. *Neuroendocrinol lett* 20: 351–64.

Stejskal, V. D. M., A. Danersund, A. Lindvall, R. Hudececk, V. Nordman, A. Yaqob, et al. 1999. Metal-specific lymphocytes: Biomarkers of sensitivity in man. *Neuroendocrinol lett* 20: 289–98.

Stern, A. 2005. A review of the studies of the cardiovascular health effects of methylmercury with consideration of their suitability for risk assessment. *Environ Res* 98(1): 133–42.

Stern, S. J. 1982. *Peru's Indian Peoples and the Challenge of Spanish Conquest: Huamanga to 1640.* Madison: University of Wisconsin Press.

Stevenson, M. 2002. Mercury from colonial silver mines poses threat in Mexico. Associated Press, November 13. www.en.com/arch.html?id=311.

Stone, R. 2003. Researchers look west to model new academy. *Science* 302: 1644.

Storelli, M. M., R. Giacominelli Stuffler, and G. O. Marcotrigiano. 2002. Total and methylmercury residues in tuna-fish from the Mediterranean Sea. *Food Additives and Contaminants* 19(8): 715–20.

The story of the laws behind the labels: Part I, 1906—Food and Drugs Act. 1981. *FDA Consumer.* www.cfsan.fda.gov/~lrd/history1.html.

The story of the laws behind the labels: Part II, 1938—The Federal Food, Drug, and Cosmetic Act. 1981. *FDA Consumer.* www.cfsan.fda.gov/~lrd/histor1a.html.

The story of the laws behind the labels: Part III, 1962—Drug Amendments. 1981. *FDA Consumer.* www.cfsan.fda.gov/~lrd/histor1b.html.

Sutton, G., and A. Chai, eds. 1997. *Hoover's Handbook of American Business: Profiles of Major U.S. Companies,* vol. 1. Austin, TX: Hoover's Business Press.

Takeuchi, T., F. M. D'Itri, P. V. Fischer, C. S. Annett, and M. Okabe. 1977. The outbreak of Minamata disease (methylmercury poisoning) in cats on northwestern Ontario reserves. *Environ Res* 13: 215–28.

Trasande, L., P. J. Landrigan, and C. Schechter. 2005. Public health and economic consequences of methylmercury toxicity to the developing brain. *Environ Health Perspect* 113: 590–96.

Truono, E. J. 1991. Response to "60 Minutes." *J Am Dent Assoc* 122(2): 10, 12, 14.

Tsuda, T. 2006. The Japanese government conceals the actual number of victims in the Minamata disease case. April 25. http://aileenarchive.or.jp/minamata_en/testimonials/index.html.

Turner, M. D., D. O. Marsh, C. E. Rubio, J. Chiriboga, C. Collazos Chiriboga, J. C. Smith, and T. W. Clarkson. 1974. Methylmercury in population eating large quantities of marine fish. I. Northern Peru. *Proc. First International Mercury Conference, Barcelona,* vol. 1, pp. 229–34. Fabrica National de Moneda y Timbre. May.

Turner, M. D., D. O. Marsh, J. C. Smith, J. B. Inglis, T. W. Clarkson, C. E. Rubio, J. Chiriboga, C. C. Chiriboga. 1980. Methylmercury in populations eating large quantities of marine fish. *Archives of Environmental Health* 35(6): 367–77.

Tyson Foods, Inc. 2004. History: Timeline. www.tyson.com/Corporate/About Tyson/History/Timeline.aspx.

Ueno, D., M. Watanabe, A. Subramanian, H. Tanaka, G. Fillmann, P. K. Lam, G. J. Zheng, M. Muchtar, H. Razak, M. Prudente, K. H. Chung, and S. Tanabe. 2005. Global pollution monitoring of polychlorinated dibenzo-p-dioxins (PCDDs), furans (PCDFs) and coplanar polychlorinated biphenyls (coplanar PCBs) using skipjack tuna as bioindicator. *Environ Pollut* 136(2): 303–13.

UK Trade and Investment. 2004. Fisheries market in the Seychelles. www.uktradeinvest.gov.uk/agriculture/seychelles2/profile/overview.shtml.

United States of America vs. Anderson Seafoods, Inc., a corporation, and Anderson Seafoods, Inc., a corporation, consolidated case with *Charles F. Anderson, an individual vs. Joseph A. Califano Jr., Secretary of Health, Education and Welfare, and Donald Kennedy, Commissioner of Food and Drugs.* United States District Court for the Northern District of Florida, Marianna Division. 447 F. Supp. 1151; Opinion 1153; February 8, 1978, U.S. Dist. Lexis 19660. MCA nos.77-0215, 77-0218 and trial transcripts of August 15, 16, 17, 18, 1977. Found in National Archives, Access #021810189, Box #3, Loc. 451927 SAN. Transcript and the following transactions were used:

- Deposition of Dr. Thomas W. Clarkson, September 17, 1977.
- Motion to prohibit filing of Dr. Clarkson's deposition unless filed under seal; no date given.
- Memorandum in support of motion to prohibit filing of deposition unless filed under seal; no date given.
- Government's memorandum in reply to Anderson's memorandum opposing the introduction of Dr. Thomas W. Clarkson's deposition in evidence; no date given.
- Government's memorandum in support of opposition to require sealing of deposition; no date given.
- Government's motion in opposition to require sealing the deposition of Dr. Clarkson, October 14, 1977.
- Anderson Seafoods, Inc.'s memorandum in opposition to government's motion for leave to introduce deposition of Dr. Thomas Clarkson in evidence, October 26, 1977.
- Judge Arnow's ruling to seal the deposition of Clarkson, October 31, 1977.

University of Rochester Medical Center. 2003. Faculty directory: G. Myers,

Department of Neurology. www.urmc.rochester.edu/neuro/fac/Myers.htm.

―――. 2007. Faculty profile: Michael Pichichero, Department of Microbiology and Immunology. www.urmc.rochester.edu/smd/mbi/faculty/pichichero .htm#Research_Focus.

U.S. Court of Appeals. 2008. *State of New Jersey et al., petitioners, vs. Environmental Protection Agency, respondent, and Utility Air Regulatory Group, et al., intervenors*, no. 05-1097. February 8.

U.S. Department of Agriculture, Food and Nutrition Service. 2006. Special supplemental nutrition program for women, infants and children (WIC): Revisions in the WIC food packages; Proposed rule. *Federal Register* 71(no. 151, August 7): 44801. www.fns.usda.gov/wic/regspublished/ foodpackagesrevisions-proposedrulepdf.pdf.

U.S. Department of Labor. 2005. The minimum wage in American Samoa. www.dol.gov/esa/whd/AS/sec5.htm.

U.S. Department of State. 2003. Peru: Profile. www.state.gov/r/pa/ei/bgn/ index.cfm?docid=2056.

―――. 2004. Post reports: Samoa. http://foia.state.gov/MMS/postrpt/ pr_view_all.asp?CntryID=126.

U.S. Department of State, Bureau of African Affairs. 2004. Background note: Seychelles. www.state.gov/r/pa/ei/bgn/6268.htm.

U.S. Department of State, Bureau of European and Eurasian Affairs. 2004. Background note: Denmark. www.state.gov/r/pa/ei/bgn/3167.htm.

U.S. Environmental Protection Agency. 1999. Potential revisions to the land disposal restrictions mercury treatment standards. *Federal Register* 64(103, May 28): 28949–28963. www.epa.gov/EPA-WASTE/1999/May/Day-28/f13659.htm.

―――. 2003. Part 2. National emission standards for hazardous air pollutants: Mercury emissions from mercury cell chlor-alkalai plants; Final rule. *Federal Register* 689(244, December 19). www.epa.gov/ttn/atw/hgcellcl/ fr19de03.pdf.

―――. 2004. Clean Air Act Amendments of 1990. Hazardous air pollutants, section 112N. www.epa.gov/air/caa/caa112.txt.

―――. 2008. Clean Air Act of 1986. www.epa.gov/air/caa/caa.txt.

―――. 2008. Clean Air Mercury Rule. February 26. www.epa.gov/camr/ basic.htm#global.

―――2008. Clear Skies Act of 2003. www.epa.gov/air/clearskies/fact2003 .html.

U.S. Food and Drug Administration. 1995. Mercury in fish: Cause for concern? *FDA Consumer*, September 1994; revised May 1995. www.cfsan .fda.gov/~acrobat/hgadv7.pdf.

―――. 1999. Letter to vaccine manufacturers regarding plans for continued use of thimerosal as a vaccine preservative. www.fda.gov/cber/ltr/thim070199.htm.

————. 2001. FDA announces advisory on methylmercury in fish. *FDA Talk Paper*, January 12. www.fda.gov/bbs/topics/answers/2001/ans01065.html.

————. 2004. What you need to know about mercury in fish and shellfish: 2004 EPA and FDA advice for women who may become pregnant, women who are pregnant, nursing mothers and children. U.S. Department of Health and Human Services and U.S. Environmental Protection Agency. March. www.cfsan.fda.gov/~dms/admehg3.html.

————. 2007. Federal Food and Drug Act of 1906 (Wiley Act). Public Law no. 59–384. 34 stst. 768 (1906). 21 U.S.C. Sec 1–15 (1934). www.fda.gov/opacom/laws/wileyact.html.

U.S. Food and Drug Administration, Department of Health and Human Services. 1998. Mercury compounds in drugs and food: Request for data and information. Docket no. 98N-1109. *Federal Register* 63(239, December 14): 68775–77. www.fda.gov/ohrms/dockets/98fr/121498e.txt.

————. 1998. Status of certain additional over-the-counter drug category II and III active ingredients. Docket nos. 75N-183F, 75N-183D, 80N-0280. *Federal Register* 63(77, April 22): 19799–802. www.GPOaccess.gov/fr/index.html.

U.S. Food and Drug Administration and U.S. Environmental Protection Agency. 2003. FDA and EPA development of a joint advisory for methylmercury-containing fish consumption for women of childbearing age and children. July 29. www.cfsan.fda.gov/~dms/mehg703c.html.

U.S. Patent and Trademark Office. 2008. Merthiolate. http://tess2.uspto.gov/bin/showfield?f=doc&state=tsfftb.4.3.

U.S. Sentencing Commission. 1995. *Report on Cocaine and Federal Sentencing Policy*, chapter 2. www.ussc.gov/crack/CHAP2.HTM.

U.S. Tuna Foundation. 2005. Congressional review finds conclusive evidence that no American is at risk from trace amounts of mercury in fish. February 16. www.tunafacts.com/press/2995/feb16.cfm.

Valentine-Thon, E., and H. Schiwara. 2003. Validity of MELISA® for metal sensitivity testing. *Neuroendocrinology Lett* 24(1–2): 57–64.

Van Wijngaarden, E., C. Beck, C. F. Shamlaye, E. Cernichiari, P. W. Davidson, G. J. Myers, and T. W. Clarkson. 2006. Benchmark concentrations for methylmercury obtained from the 9-year follow-up of the Seychelles Child Development Study. U.S. Environmental Protection Agency. *Neurotoxicology* 27(5): 702–9.

Varekamp, J. C., B. Kreulen, M. R. Buchholtz ten Brink, and E. L. Mecray. 2003. Mercury contamination chronologies from Connecticut wetlands and Long Island Sound sediments. *Environ Geol* 43: 268–82.

Via, C. S., P. Nguyen, F. Niculescu, J. Papadimitriou, D. Hoover, and E. Silbergeld. 2003. Low dose exposure to inorganic mercury accelerates disease and mortality in acquired murine lupus. *Environ Health Perspect* 111: 1273–77.

Virtanen, J. K., S. Voutilainen, T. H. Rissanen, J. Mursu, T. Tuomainen, M. J. Korhonen, et al. 2005. Mercury, fish oils, and risk of acute coronary events and cardiovascular disease, coronary heart disease, and all-cause mortality in men in eastern Finland. *Arterioscler Thromb Vasc Biol* 25: 228–33.

Vogl, A. 1950. The discovery of the organic mercurial diuretics. *Am Heart J* 39: 881–83.

Walker, M. 1996. *The President We Deserve: Bill Clintion, His Rise, Falls, and Comebacks.* New York: Crown.

Watson, A. 2002. The very model of a modern Iraqi dissident. *Science* 298(5598): 1543.

Wheatley, B., A. Barbeau, T. W. Clarkson, and L. W. Lapham. 1979. Methylmercury poisoning in Canadian Indians: The elusive diagnosis. *Canadian J Neur Sci* 6(4): 417–22.

Wijngaarden, E. V., C. Beck, C. F. Shamlaye, E. Cernichiari, P. W. Davidson, G. J. Myers, and T. W. Clarkson. 2006. Benchmark concentrations for methylmercury obtained from the 9-year follow-up of the Seychelles Child Development Study. *Neurotoxicology* 27(5): 702–9.

World Culture Encyclopedia. Africa/Middle East: Kurds: Religion and expressive culture. www.everyculture.com/Africa-Middle-East/Kurds.html. 2007.

World Health Organization. 1972. Technical Report Series no. 505. FAO Nutrition Meetings Report Series no. 51. Evaluation of certain food additives and the contaminants mercury, lead, and cadmium. Sixteenth report of the Joint FAO/WHO food additives series 52. Methylmercury addendum 2004. Switzerland. Available: www.inchem.org/documents/jecfa/jecmono/v52je23.htm#esd. accessed 10/17/2007. Expert Committee on Food Additives, Geneva, April 4–12.

———. 1990. Environmental Health Criteria 101: Methylmercury. International Programme on Chemical Safety, Geneva. www.inchem.org/documents/ehc/ehc/ehc101.htm#SubSectionNumber:9.1.1.

———. 2000. WHO Food Additives Series 44: Safety evaluation of certain food additives and contaminants. Prepared by the fifty-third meeting of the Joint FAO/WHO Expert Committee on Food Additives (JECFA), Geneva. www.inchem.org/documents/jecfa/jecmono/v44jec13.htm.

———. 2004. WHO Food Additives Series 52: Methylmercury addendum. www.inchem.org/documents/jecfa/jecmono/v52je23.htm#esd.

Wyngaarden, J. B., L. H. Smith, and J. C. Bennet. 1992. *Cecil Textbook of Medicine*, 19th ed. John Dyson, ed. Philadelphia: W.B. Saunders, pp. 2364, 2374.

Yokoo, E. M., J. G. Valente, L. Grattan, S. L. Schmidt, I. Platt, and E. K. Silbergeld. 2003. Low level methylmercury exposure affects neuropsychological functioning in adults. *Environ Health* 2: 8.

Index

Note: page numbers followed by "n" refer to endnotes.

About the Author

JANE M. HIGHTOWER, MD is a Board Certified Internal Medicine physician in San Francisco, California. She published a landmark study that brought the issue of mercury in seafood to national attention. She continues to publish scientific papers and give lectures on the subject. She has appeared on numerous television and radio programs to discuss the concerns about the mercury that is prevalent in the fish we consume.

About Island Press

Since 1984, the nonprofit Island Press has been stimulating, shaping, and communicating the ideas that are essential for solving environmental problems worldwide. With more than 800 titles in print and some 40 new releases each year, we are the nation's leading publisher on environmental issues. We identify innovative thinkers and emerging trends in the environmental field. We work with world-renowned experts and authors to develop cross-disciplinary solutions to environmental challenges.

Island Press designs and implements coordinated book publication campaigns in order to communicate our critical messages in print, in person, and online using the latest technologies, programs, and the media. Our goal: to reach targeted audiences—scientists, policymakers, environmental advocates, the media, and concerned citizens—who can and will take action to protect the plants and animals that enrich our world, the ecosystems we need to survive, the water we drink, and the air we breathe.

Island Press gratefully acknowledges the support of its work by the Agua Fund, Inc., Annenberg Foundation, The Christensen Fund, The Nathan Cummings Foundation, The Geraldine R. Dodge Foundation, Doris Duke Charitable Foundation, The Educational Foundation of America, Betsy and Jesse Fink Foundation, The William and Flora Hewlett Foundation, The Kendeda Fund, The Forrest and Frances Lattner Foundation, The Andrew W. Mellon Foundation, The Curtis and Edith Munson Foundation, Oak Foundation, The Overbrook Foundation, the David and Lucile Packard Foundation, The Summit Fund of Washington, Trust for Architectural Easements, Wallace Global Fund, The Winslow Foundation, and other generous donors.

The opinions expressed in this book are those of the author(s) and do not necessarily reflect the views of our donors.